THE RE-EMERGENCE OF TAMA-RE SMAI TAUI AFRIKAN

A Practical Guide to
Wellbeing Through Smai Posture,
Breath and Meditation

Pablo M Imani

The Re-emergence of Tama-re Smai Taui Afrikan Yoga

A Practical Guide to Wellbeing Through Smai Posture, Breath and Meditation

Copyright © 2008, 2021 Pablo M Imani

Health and Wellbeing

All Rights Reserved. No part of this book may be reproduced in any manner whatsoever, or stored in any information storage system, or transmitted in any form or by any means; electronic, mechanical, photocopying, recording, or otherwise, without prior written consent of the publisher, except in the case of brief quotations with proper reference, embodied in articles and reviews.

Printed in the United Kingdom

ISBN 978-1-8381797-0-0

Photographs by Pablo M Imani, Moud Imhotep, Thomas Gerdy Mahrenholz, Calise Cleghorn and Karina Al Piaro

Published by Pimay Publishing

Editorial Production: The Editor's Chair

DEDICATION

To my deities in the flesh, the children who blessed me: Kha'mara (Black Sun), Nefertem (Beautiful Completion), and Amenta (Keeper of The Secrets). You are so good for me; you have expanded me and continue to do so, may you find your true paths.

To the Smai students and Afrikan Yogis everywhere, come home.

To those who are awakening, welcome, let's work together.

CONTENTS

Acknowledgements - 2

Foreword - 3

Preface - 4

INTRODUCTION - 5

AFRIKAN BACKGROUND OF YOGA

Afrikan Yoga? - 15
Hatha or Hat Hor - 18
The Foundations of Afrikan Yoga - 21

MENTAL HEALTH

The Radiance of a Great Master Teacher's Tool - 32
Tehuti - 36
The 9 Principles of Tehuti Related to Yoga - 38

Mental; Correspondence; Vibration; Polarity; Rhythm; Cause and Effect; Gender; Growth; Breath

SPIRITUAL HEALTH

Sekhem Spark of Life - 48
Nine to the 9th Power - 52
The Ennead of Afrikan Yoga 9 Neteru - 55
The 9 Principles of the Human Being - 61
The 9 Purposes of Smai/Afrikan Yoga - 65

Emancipation/Freedom; Action; Knowledge; Power; Love; Transcendence; Wisdom; Joy; Truth

HEALTH & WELLBEING

Afrikan Seats of Light 9 Arushaat/Chakras - 71
The Connection of Arushaat to Melanin

Personalities of Unbalanced and Balanced Arushaat/Energy Centres - 76
Hikau Word-Sound and Power... The Science of Sound Healing - 81
Afrikan Yoga and its Benefits - 90

Hudu; The Eye of Re; Neck Rolls; Sitting Sanyaat for Meditation; Hand Positions

Patarugshil-Re; The Journey of Re - 119

Hand Positions - 121
Meditation - 125
Suggestions for a Beneficial Practice - 128

Time & Patience; Nutrition; Drink Water; Deep Breathing;
Rest & Relaxation; Sleep; Positive Affirmation; Epilogue

Bibliography and Recommended Reading - 142
Glossary and Definitions - 143

Reconnect to The Source

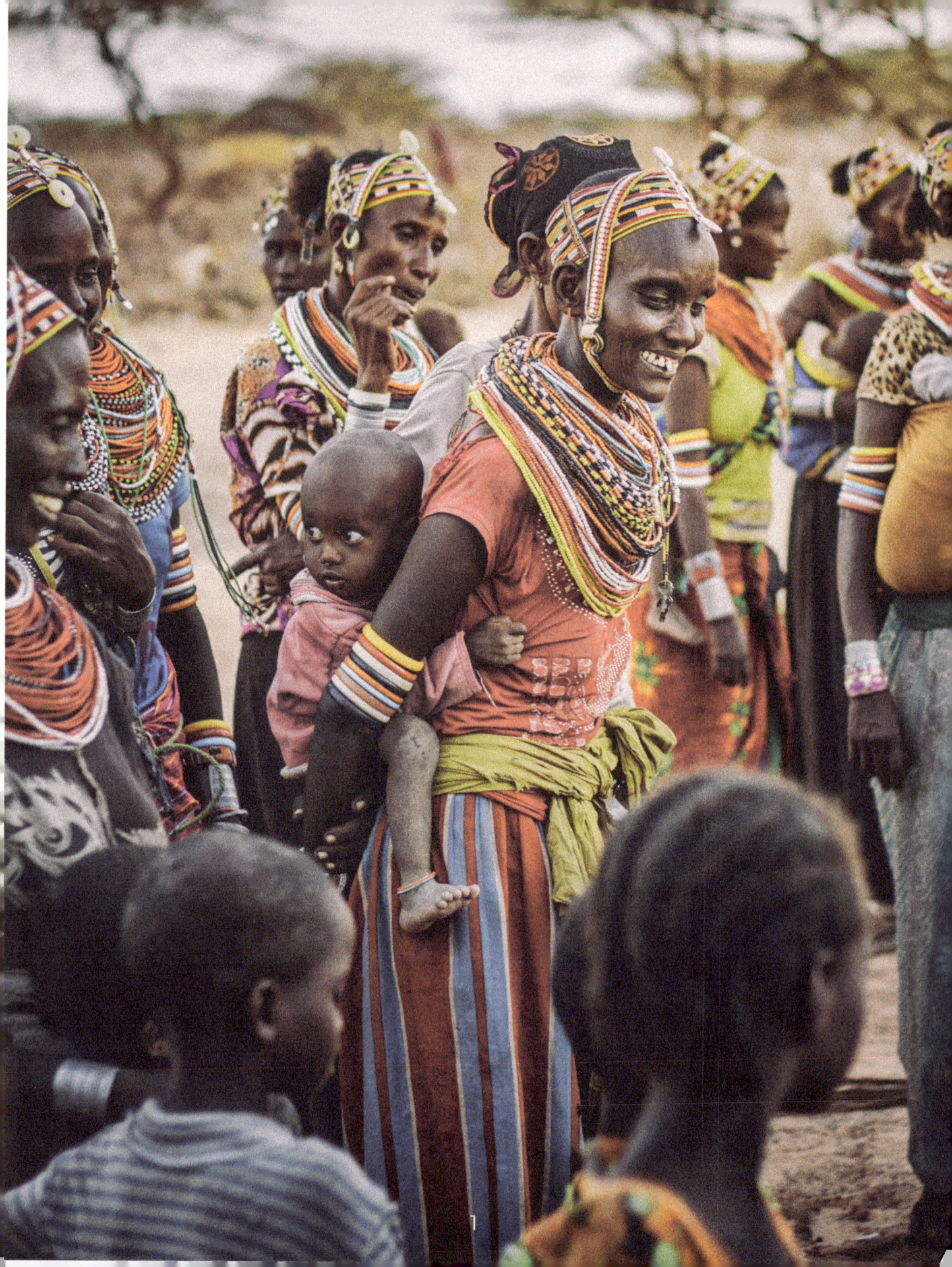

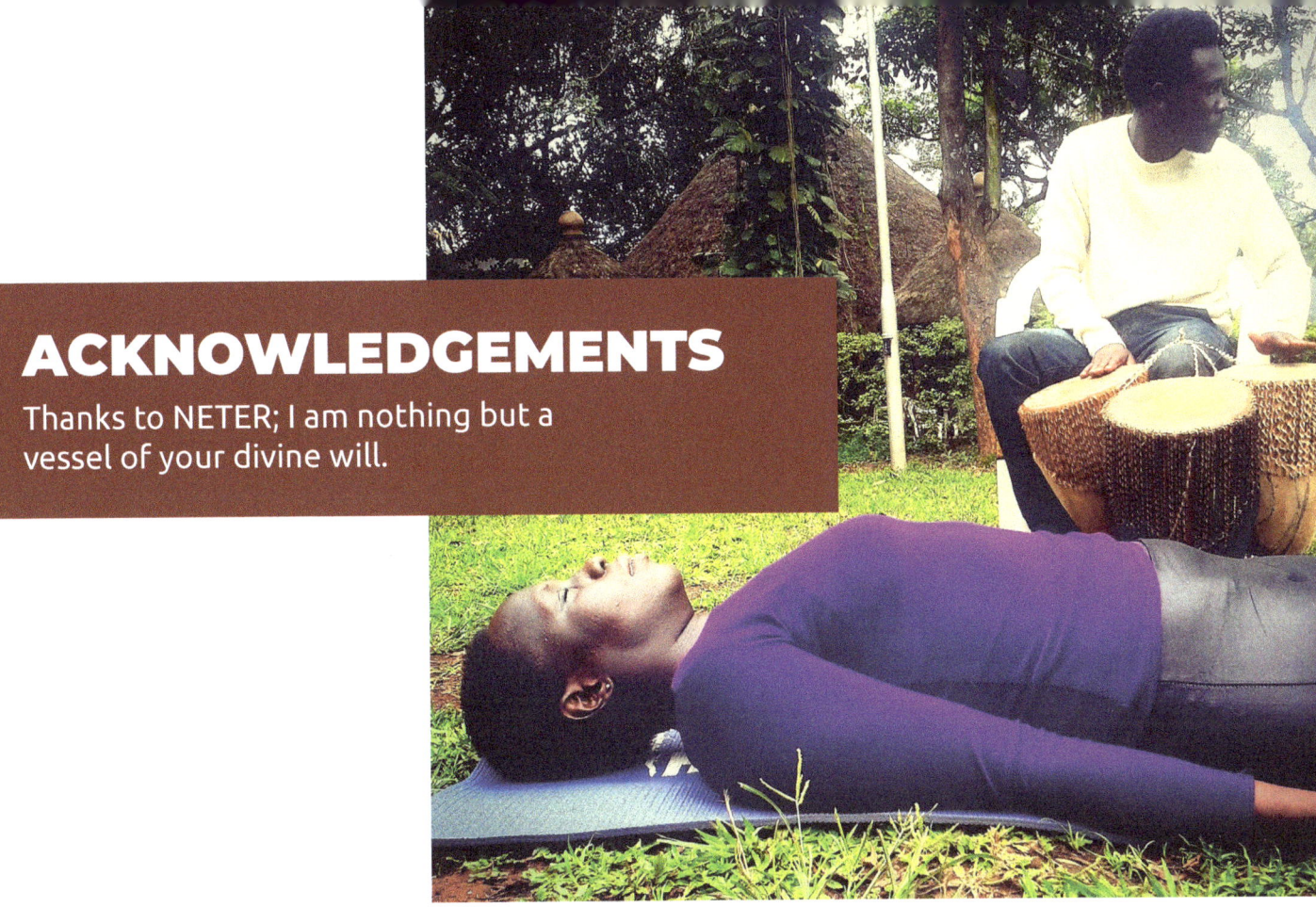

ACKNOWLEDGEMENTS
Thanks to NETER; I am nothing but a vessel of your divine will.

The Neteru cosmic forces of nature, Orishas, and my divine and righteous Ancestors, ancient and modern, I thank you each and every day with all my being. You strengthen my body, soul, and spirit. You reside in my being because when I look within, all I see is your boundless blackness. When I look without, all I see is your supreme manifestations. Thank you truly for the personification of Smai Afrikan Yoga as a science of reconnecting and the personification of this book.

To The Supreme Grand Master Teacher Amunnubi Ruakh Ptah…

Thank you for accepting me as a student in the Ancient Mystic Order of Melchizedek and the Ancient Egyptian Order. Since the day we met, your enthusiasm and humility have always struck a resounding chord for me. Thank you for raising me from the mentally dead and inspiring me with your words, deeds, and tireless work. You wrote over 360 books and planted seeds in thousands, which signifies Tehuti incarnate. You showed me that it was possible to incarnate our great blood seed ancestors, Pa Neters, here and now. You made terms like 'Right Knowledge' common amongst Africans in the Diaspora. You are the A'aferti (Pharaoh) in this day and time. You taught me not to be afraid to be different, to accept my opposing natures and unify them (Smai Tawi). Your spirit cannot be contained for it is here with us around the globe. This work is, indeed, a testament to your teaching, which I have attempted to disseminate in the way I was guided to do.

FOREWORD

Over the years yoga interest and economy has grown astronomically. It used by global companies in advertising and is revered the world over. The increase in the number of people ready to reconnect to the source, with the need to go deeper into self and release the blocked and locked tensions of old, is brimming and flowing in every corner of the planet.

Many prophecies and predictions by indigenous cultures to what is coming and what is here, awakens our core like a galactic clock aligning us to the reality of existence. The timeless wisdom of yoga and Ancient Africa is a forerunner to the coming paradigm shifts that we are presently experiencing, teaching us to trust spirit, connect to life, run with nature, delve into the essence of our being, and connect to the source.

Afrikan Yoga Smai Taui has emerged in this timely fashion out of the Nile Valley the land of Hapi, as the breath of Ancient African culture, a balm to replenish our mind, body, and soul in this Kali Yuga age of tension and stress.

The teaching of balance between the upper and lower natures, spirit and body are invaluably rich and potent. Smai Taui is the Integrating elevating conscious wisdom of the Ancient African lifting those who engage into higher states of being.

Pablo Imani's book, Afrikan Yoga, and his works in the areas of yoga promoting a system of healing and self-cultivation from an African perspective, is not only an imperative for Africans and those of African descent, but for the entire world community. This science is long-awaited and Pablo has answered the call of the ancients. He, in turn, invites you to partake of this transformative, emotionally cleansing, life-giving system that assists you to regain your wholeness and wellness as well as to reconnect you to the source.

Let these pages inspire you to move beyond internal barriers and enrich you with spirit. Allow them to raise your awareness of the bountiful wisdom teachings of Tama-re Smai Taui.

Professor Benjamin Zephaniah
Author of Kung Fu Trip
and Too Black Too Strong

PREFACE

Yoga is on the rise and its popularity is due to the need to de-stress in an ever-growing stressful environment. There are countless amounts of classes all over the UK. The British Wheel of Yoga, the largest yoga organization in the UK, has a network of over 3,000 qualified registered teachers, not to mention many more that are registered with other organizations. I took up Chinese yoga, commonly referred to as 'Tai Chi', to help alleviate my back problems. However, it was the practice of Afrikan yoga that healed my back pain within a week of steady practice. It proved to me that the system was a cultural practice, which was also directly linked to one's body type and that all healing systems were specifically created by and for the culture and the people (body type) of that culture. This is more accurately termed 'Ethnomedicine' in reference to Dr Llaila O Afrika and Dr Jewel Pookrum.

This also taught me that my genetic make-up has a spiritual component that will grow or deplete with whatever I take on board as a spiritual path/practice.

Afrikans who seek in their own language and symbolism will powerfully bring peace to this planet by first seeking it in themselves.

This book is a stimulant, using scriptures, for example, **Coming Forth by Day; The Husia: Sacred Wisdom of Ancient Egypt** written by Nubians. Some of the scriptures complement and predate the Hindu, Buddhist texts. This is not to negate Taoist or Hindu texts, which I have read and gained valuable food for thought and wisdom from. In this piece of work, I have also applied The Sacred Wisdom of Tehuti to Afrikan Yoga and the principles found therein as well as offered a practical guide to Smai postures, breath and meditation.

"Follow the footsteps of your ancestors for the mind is trained through knowledge. Behold, their words endure in books. Open and read them and follow their wise counsel for one who is taught becomes skilled. Do not be evil for kindness is good. Make the memory of you last through the love of you."

The Book of Kheti, the Husia, Sacred Wisdom of Ancient Egypt

INTRODUCTION

TAMA-RE SMAI
Awakening Soul through

Earth, Water & Fire union

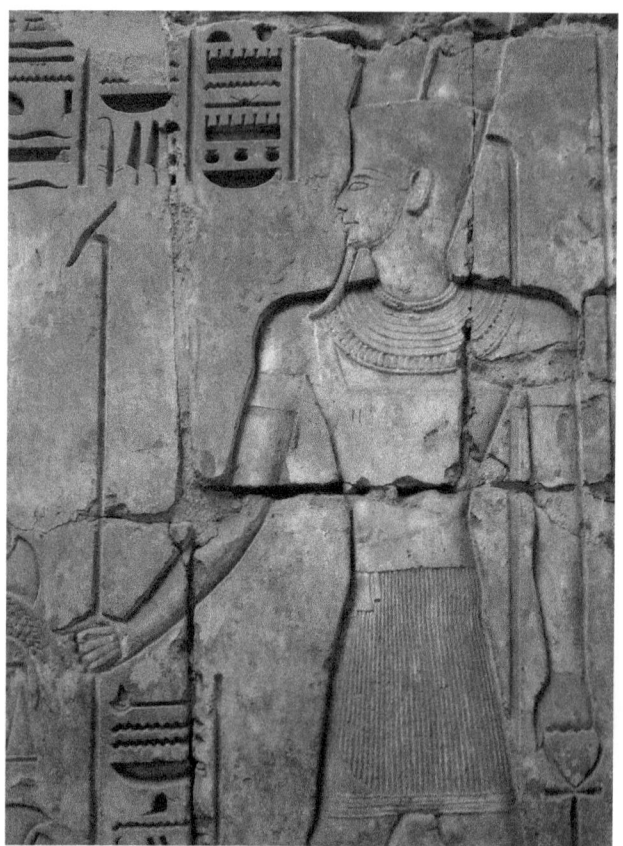 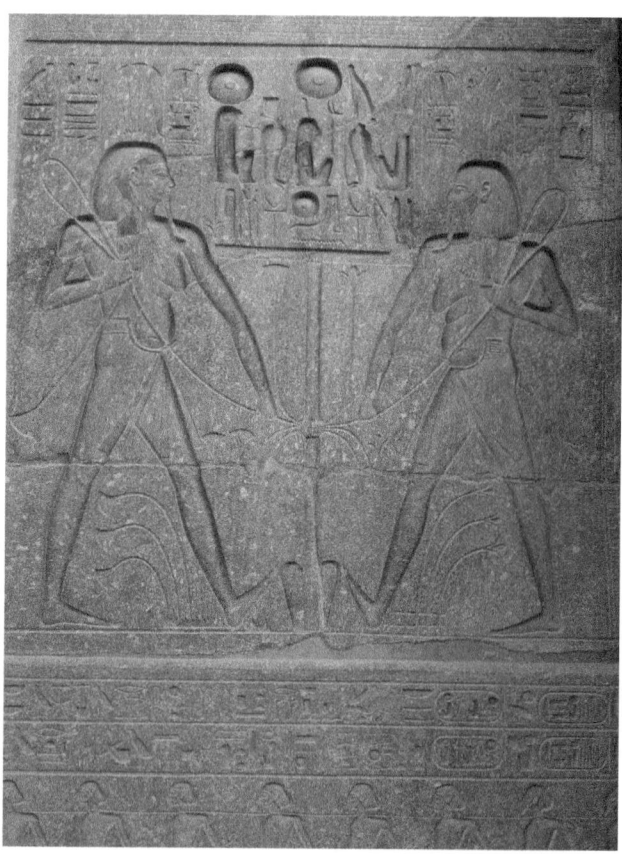

One of the most difficult things to do is to attempt to convince someone that what they have been led to believe all their lives is false, that the information they have built their businesses on or their leisure activities, which they have invested in over the years, developing sentimental strings and even building their family unit, is not only wrong but is more insidiously a lie.

In reading this book, I merely ask you to read with an open mind. Take time to meditate and make the connection with your Ancient Afrikan ancestors now miscalled Egyptians. They will provide you with the wisdom you seek in making the choices in regards to your health, your way of life, 'Ba Tarug', and the reconnection to the power source in which you are seeking.

> "Truth alone is eternal and immutable; truth is the first blessing; but truth is not and cannot be on earth; everything has matter on it, clothed with a corporeal form subject to change, to alteration. The things of earth are but appearances and imitations of truth; they are what the picture is to reality."
>
> Tehuti

The Process of Healing

People of Afrika – "A free Ka" – are led to believe that they did not originate anything. All that you see around you, Afrikans had nothing to do with it. Often times I hear an Afrikan individual say, "Well, I can do yoga, Zen, Buddhism, Shinto, and Celtic stuff because I'm universal." I am aware that Afrikans sometimes feel the need to be inclusive. Now is the time to pry your eyes open and view what scientists have already proven, that all came from Afrika. Tama-re and the first world civilisations started in Afrika. All these systems that we wish to be included in, are born out of Africa anyway, right? So why are Afrikans not sticking to their thing or even trying to find out what their thing is? Afrikans the world over have settled and submerged in a watered-down, warped and poisoned version of ways of being. Afrikans have been bred out of their minds and their culture. Afrikans are led to partake of all other cultures appropriations of what Ethiopians, Nubians, Kushites and Afrikans originated. Racism does exist yet we, 'The modern-day Afrikan', keep it in existence by our very thoughts and attitudes towards one another, their local communities, and the world. Afrikans must realise that they no longer should be led by anyone.

Afrikans live on a day-to-day basis with a constant victim mentality. Not realising that they are powerful enough to change the state of affairs in their lives and the affairs of this planet, they settle for states of illusions. Our reality is re-created daily by what we think and how we think. Afrikans can achieve what they will when they see and feel the joy of whom and what they are today as well as the pride of what they once were.

Now because I am pro-Afrikan does not mean I hate other races of people and I'm writing because I have an axe to grind, chip on my shoulder, or just plainly ignorantly verbally abusing others. For those who are reading this book, this is not my intention. The abuse has got to stop and the healing must begin.

This healing process often starts by facing what hurts and what appears to be discomforting so if you are a European or Asian practitioner reading this book, you too must heal and that means having an awareness of what your ancestors and peers and maybe you yourself are doing to the darker peoples of this world by not facing up to the reality of your past and living off shame. Face that truth and develop your humanity to bring consciousness to this planet by working through Ma'at (Truth Justice Balance).

Let all the people of this planet work together for the sake of the planet and let the truth prevail. No more lies, no more cover-ups. Truth is truth.

The Language in this book

Egypt had many dialects throughout its civilization. The dialects changed over periods of time owing to the various invasions that eventually caused Egypt and, indeed, the entire African continent to decline. Some of these dialects are completely lost, which is evident as Arabic is the main language of modern-day Egypt. The language I used is called Nuwaupic, as was introduced to me by my spiritual preceptor, Amunnubi Ruakh Ptah, this is the language not of the pharaohs or the general population but the language of Pa Neteru. A language whose origin was of the pre-dynastic period, that supposedly died out during the Greek and Roman invasions around 30BC and was replaced with Coptic. The western and European writers make claims that this old language was lost until a French man named Jean Francois Champollion deciphered the hieroglyphs in 1822. The claim is that he was the first to decipher the language correctly; this is a bold statement, as we now know that European translations of Afrikan languages and culture are not devoid of subjectivity and European cultural bias with its emphasis on entertainment value.

Would an Englishman accept a modern-day African linguist deciphering the old Anglo-Saxon or Germanic language and have that as the basis of their learning about that culture in that time for their school children?

This is not impossible, however; Afrikans do have an option right now in regard to the ancient language of Egypt and that is Amunnubi Ruakh Ptah, a Sudanese by birth and linguistic speaker of 19 languages, who reintroduced the lost language called Nuwaupic or Nuwaubic prior to the invasions. We also have several Afrikan scholars around the world who have deciphered what is known as the 'Medu Neter' sacred writings for themselves. They have a clearer insight as they do not use just intellect but genetic memory.

Nuwaupic

This language, Nuwaupic, appears in Ancient Sumer (Babylon), also called Cuneiform today. The cuneiform gave birth to Phoenician, Accadian, Chaldean, Ugaritic, Aramic, Hebraic, and Syriac Ashuric Arabic. This is the language you will see and hear throughout this book. Nuwaupic can appear as a script or as a glyph. It is basically spoken in tones vibrating from the diaphragm, which stimulate the spiritual seats in the body and is used to re-align human beings to The Guardians, Pa Neteru. I hope that Afrikan Yoga will be practised by Afrikans on the continent and around the globe using Afrikan languages that the individual is familiar with. Afrikan languages often use full vowel intonation and the diaphragm, which is why Afrikans have deeper, melodic voices, and the ability to sing the way they do. So all Afrikans can easily practice Smai science with the use of Xiosa, Twi, Ga, Fanti, Igbo, Zulu, Mende, Wolof, Fulani, Amharic, and Swahili etc., languages used presently. Nature's elements, Neteru, Orisha etc., remain the same for all of us.

As long as Afrikans begin to value what is theirs, we will take this Smai- Afrikan Yoga, one of our many sciences, back to where it belongs in our everyday live-ity.

I have used the term 'Africa' spelt purposely 'Afrika' or 'A Free Ka' (a free spirit) on promotional materials and even to short cut the description of what I do to perspective students. I have chosen to redefine the word Africa as this word universally means a downtrodden separated people and this piece of writing in no way wants to promote this present world view of Solar (sun) people.

You may notice that many are comfortable with the title 'Africa', which derives from the Arabic word Farraq 'to divide'. The word 'Africa' has been said to have various sources, all of which are foreign to the present day nine ether solar beings who reside on the Mother Father continent, at the centre of the world. Ethiopians, Tamareans, Nubian Kushite peoples that means all nine ether solar beings descended from an ancient and cosmic heritage.

Af Re Ka is a definition that I explored as the 'Af' is short for Aferti meaning Pharaoh. 'Re' represents the sun specifically and The Most High, and 'Ka' means spirit. Afrikans are truly sun peoples of a divine nature and are the descendants of Re. This is not myth, this is by blood lineage as these beings, 'The Neteru', at one time walked this earth and that's why there is a genetic memory, restlessness, an affinity with nature; a deep love and compassion that only a 'being' of high culture could emanate. This is why Afrikans are so hard to destroy and why they are feared by those who have a low-level egotistic mind. This vague remanence of high culture is expandable; it can be nurtured and grown. The Neteru left us clues and guides having foreseen their demise. They knew that at some point we would lose our way and left us these to help us to find our way back. However, in the Yogic tradition the Smai practitioner is a free-spirited being and what Afrikans call for the world over is to be what we all once were and that is to be free. We cannot be truly free unless we are free in body, mind and spirit. Afrikan Yoga frees the spirit by working through the body first. So A Free Ka (spirit) is the definition I coined and use intermittently with Afrika. So do not look at this word merely as a continent or place but see it as a state of mind and spirit.

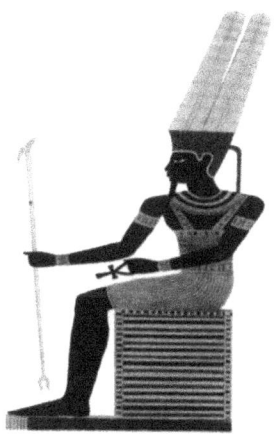

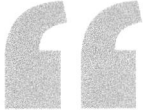

Lift up the self by the self, and don't let the self weaken, for the self is the self's only friend, and the self is the self's only foe.

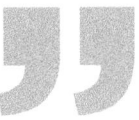

The Grand Master Dr Malachi Z York
The Book of Urim and Thummim

The Earliest Known Inhabitants of India...

The Harappan

The Harappan civilization spreads all over India; 1,000 sites have been uncovered by archaeologists; the two main cities being Mohenjo-Daro and Harappa, dating as far back as 3000 B.C.

The Harappans flourished along the river 'Indus', as did the Sumerians along the Tigris Euphrates and the Khemitians along the Nile.

They farmed and cultivated cotton. They had their own script and even though they were mainly pastoralist they were also builders who had drainage and sewage systems in their homes and throughout their settlements. The Harappans even formed bodily decorations using beads, copper, silver, gold, and bronze. They created necklaces and bangles.

The Harappans have been favoured by scholars to be the earliest inhabitants of India and often seem to be used as a description of the Dravidians; even European and Indian scholars find them to be Black and Africoid.

Those of us who have looked very closely at India's population, history, and culture find it to be very mixed.

> "In India... there are also traces of intermingling with the Negro race to which part of the darkness of the skin so widely prevalent in India may be attributed".

Elliot Smith, Human History, pp. 134-145
London, 1934

Marco Polo described the inhabitants of India as black and adorned with massive gold bracelets and strings of rare and precious gems. They had temples and priests. Vasco de Gama while circumnavigating the globe found the inhabitants black. (From the book: The Wonderful Ethiopians of the Ancient Cushite Empire, Chapter 15, The Civilization of India.)

Harrapans

The people about whom I have been speaking are descendants of Cushites; they are a combination of two Black races, the Black Negroid (resembling Africans) and the Black Australoid (resembling Australian Aborigines. India is known to have some of the purest Black people on earth. These include the Black Dalit/Untouchables, who were kept segregated and isolated for thousands of years by the 'Indo-Europeans', who invaded India from North-Eastern Europe. The brown-skinned to fair-skinned people with features similar to Middle Eastern and Iranian people are of Caucasian origins and live mainly in the North West of India.

The Ethiopian Dravidians

The Dravidians in ethnic type are Ethiopian and are the race of India from which her civilization originated. Megathenes said that the natives of India and Ethiopia were not much different in complexion or feature. Dravidians are short like the race of the Mediterranean called Iberians and the Chaldeans. Their complexions are black or very dark. Their hair is plentiful and crispy. Their heads are elongated with the nose very broad. They occupy the oldest geological formation of India. They are descendants of that race of Black men with short woolly hair that were the primitive inhabitants of Ancient Media, Susiana, and Persia, mentioned repeatedly in the Iranian legends, and whose faces look out at us from the sculptures of Babylon and Nineveh. Dravidian is spoken by 46 million Indians, not including the numerous uncultivated hill tribes and retired communities. A form of speech similar to it is spoken in Baluchistan, which originally was Kushite.

Concept of the Dravidian Race

The identification of the Dravidian people as a separate race arose from the realization by 19th-century Western scholars that there existed a group of languages spoken by people in the south of India, which were completely unrelated to the Indo-Aryan languages prevalent in the north of the country. Because of this, it was supposed that the generally darker-skinned Dravidian speakers constituted a genetically distinct race. This notion corresponded to European belief of the time, according to which darker-skinned peoples were more "primitive" than the light-skinned whites. Accordingly, Dravidians were envisaged as primitive early inhabitants of India who had been partially displaced and subordinated by Aryans. The term Dravidian is taken from the Sanskrit "drÇvida", meaning "Southern". It was adopted following the publication of Robert Caldwell's Comparative Grammar of the Dravidian or South-Indian Family of Languages (1856); a publication which established the language grouping as one of the major language groups of the world. (http://en.wikipedia.org)

Speaking of languages, in his researched piece called the 'Cultural Unity of African Languages', Clyde A. Winter explains that, "Dravidian languages are predominately spoken in southern India and Sri Lanka. There are around 125 million Dravidian speakers. These languages are genetically related to African languages. The Dravidians are remnants of the ancient Black population who occupied most of Ancient Asia and Europe."

Clyde further informs us of the unity between Ancient Indian languages and African languages by making cultural and linguistic comparisons. The Dravidians have maintained their Ancient African heritage. There are numerous affinities between Dravidian and Black African culture and languages. As in Africa, the Dravidians built there both small and large vessels from a single log or planks tied together. This method of boat construction has been common in Africa since the rise of Ancient Egypt and continues today in East Africa, Chad, and along the Niger River. In both Africa and Dravidian India, the people were organized into various "caste" or corporations. Many of the corporations such as that of the blacksmiths in Africa and India have corresponding names e.g., Wolof Kamara and Telugu Kamara. There are similarities in agricultural technique in Africa and India. For example, both groups used the hoe for tilling the ground, manuring the ground to fertilize crops, terracing irrigation, and canal building. There are also affinities in animal husbandry and even the names of animals. For example, Wolof xar: 'sheep'; Brahui (Dravidian) xar: 'ram' and 'cow'; Wolof nag, Serere nak Tamil naku: 'a female buffalo'; and Tulu naku: 'heifer'. There are also similarities between the Dravidian and African religions. For example, both groups held a common interest in the cult of the Serpent (Kundalini) and believed in a Supreme God, who lived in a place of peace and tranquillity. There are also affinities between the names of many gods including Amun/Amma and Murugan. Murugan, the Dravidian god of the mountains, parallels a common god in East Africa worshipped by 25 ethnic groups called Murungu, the god who resides in the mountains. In addition among the Ali tiravitar, the system of inheritance passes from the uncle to his nephews, instead of to his sons (maru makkal Tayam) as in Africa. And in both South India and the Western Sudan of Africa, the dead were buried in terra cotta jars.

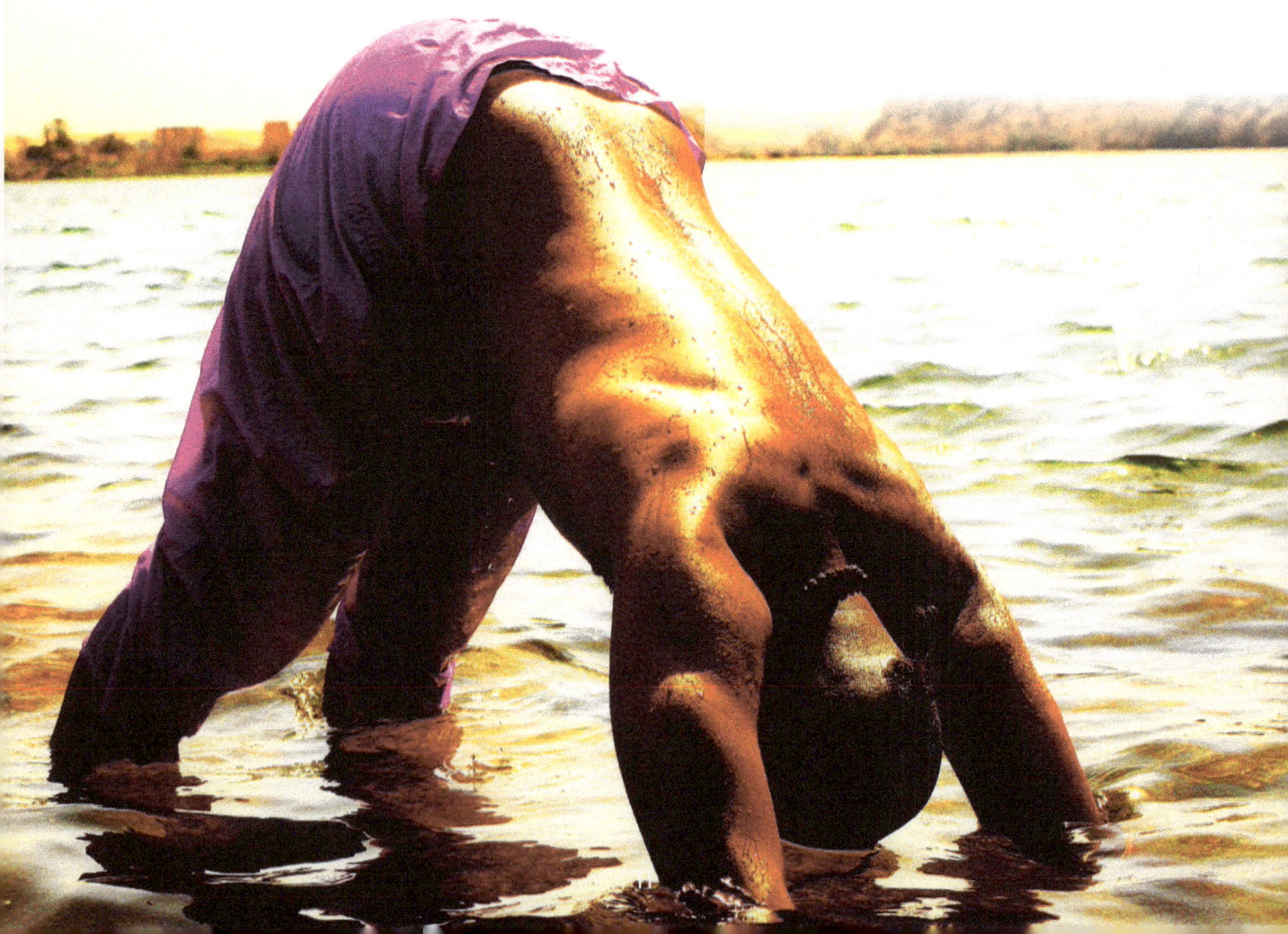

Lower Ancient Egypt

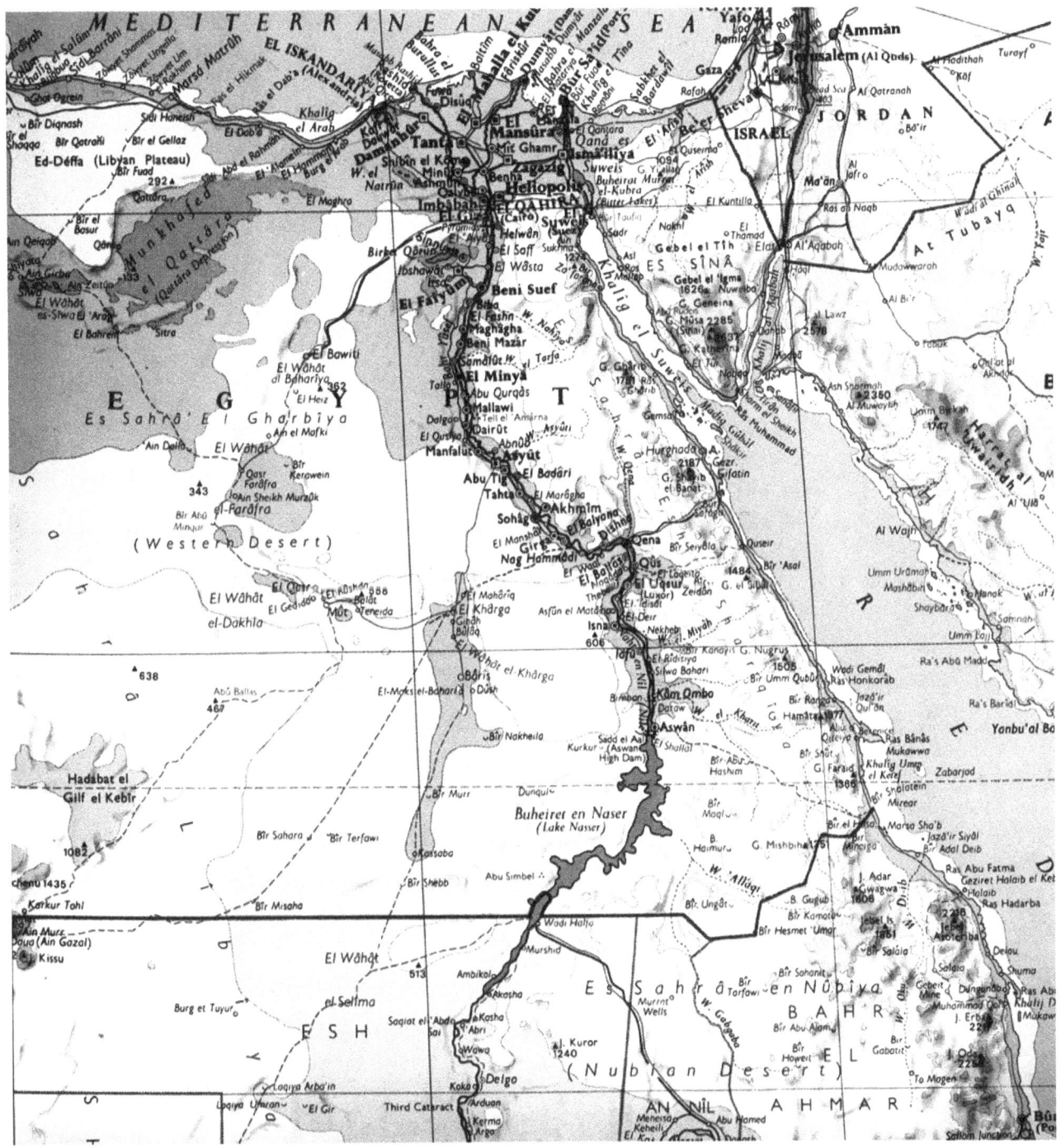

Ancient Egypt/Khemet spread from the North of present-day Afrika down to Kenya, Uganda, and Zimbabwe.

Dr Zacharias Thundy of Northern Michigan University believes that the Dravidians may have left Nubia after Senefru (c.2613 B.C.) conquered Nubia. Senefru's raid caused much destruction and may have encouraged many Kushites to flee Nubia for safe areas of settlement.

Calumet testifies that from ancient accounts and from all recent research, culture and civilization spread into Egypt from the south and especially from Meroe. Egypt, ruled at first by several contemporary kings, was finally united into one great kingdom. Priesthood seemed to have governed the land. The head of the state was a priest. The sacred books of the Hindu speak of an "Old Race", (Tar-ites, Twa, and the Nubuns ancestors to the Tama-reans/Kemetians Ancient Afrikans) that came down from Upper Egypt and peopled the delta. They mentioned the Mountains of the Moon and the Nile flowing through Barabra. Herodotus says in his second book, "They say that in the time of Menes/Narmer (first Dynasty) all Egypt except the district of Thebes was a morass, and that no part of the land now existing below Lake Myris was then above water. To this place from the sea is seven days passage up the river..." Diodorus Siculus (author of Library of World History) says in Book Three, "The Ethiopians say that the Egyptians are a colony drawn out of them by Osiris; and that Egypt was formerly no part of the continent but a sea at the beginning of the world, and that it was afterwards made land by the river Nile."

Upper Ancient Egypt

Diaspora. The original culture of Egypt came from what was called Upper Egypt at the origin of the Nile, Uganda, Tanzania, on through Kenya, Ethiopia, and Sudan. This begun in the Congo before borders, where the Twa or Pthar-ites reside and this culture spread throughout all of Afrika and indeed on to other parts of the world.

The All is I am
"I am the Universe and the Universe is I
I am balanced, graceful and beautiful.
The Universe is balanced, graceful and beautiful.
I am the Universe and the Universe is I".

Khonsu Sekhem Ptah

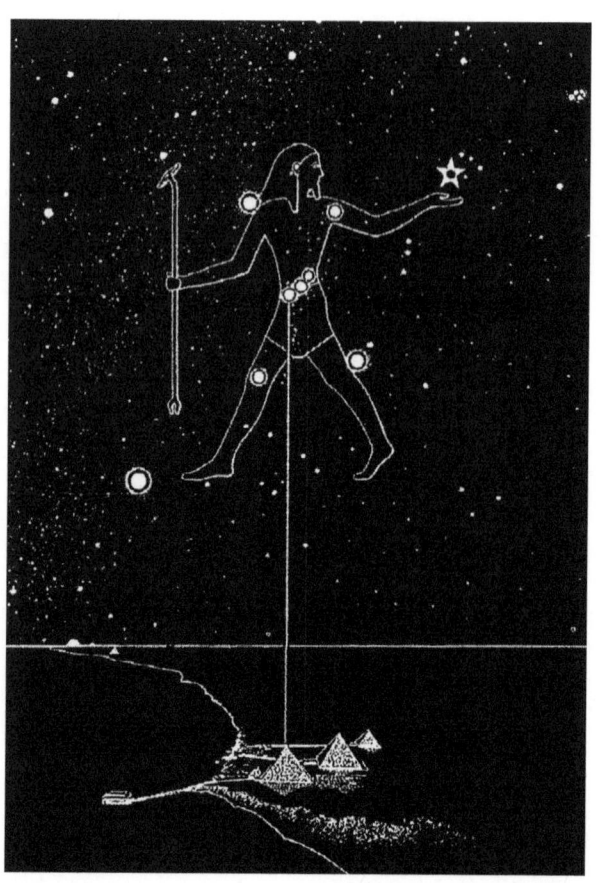

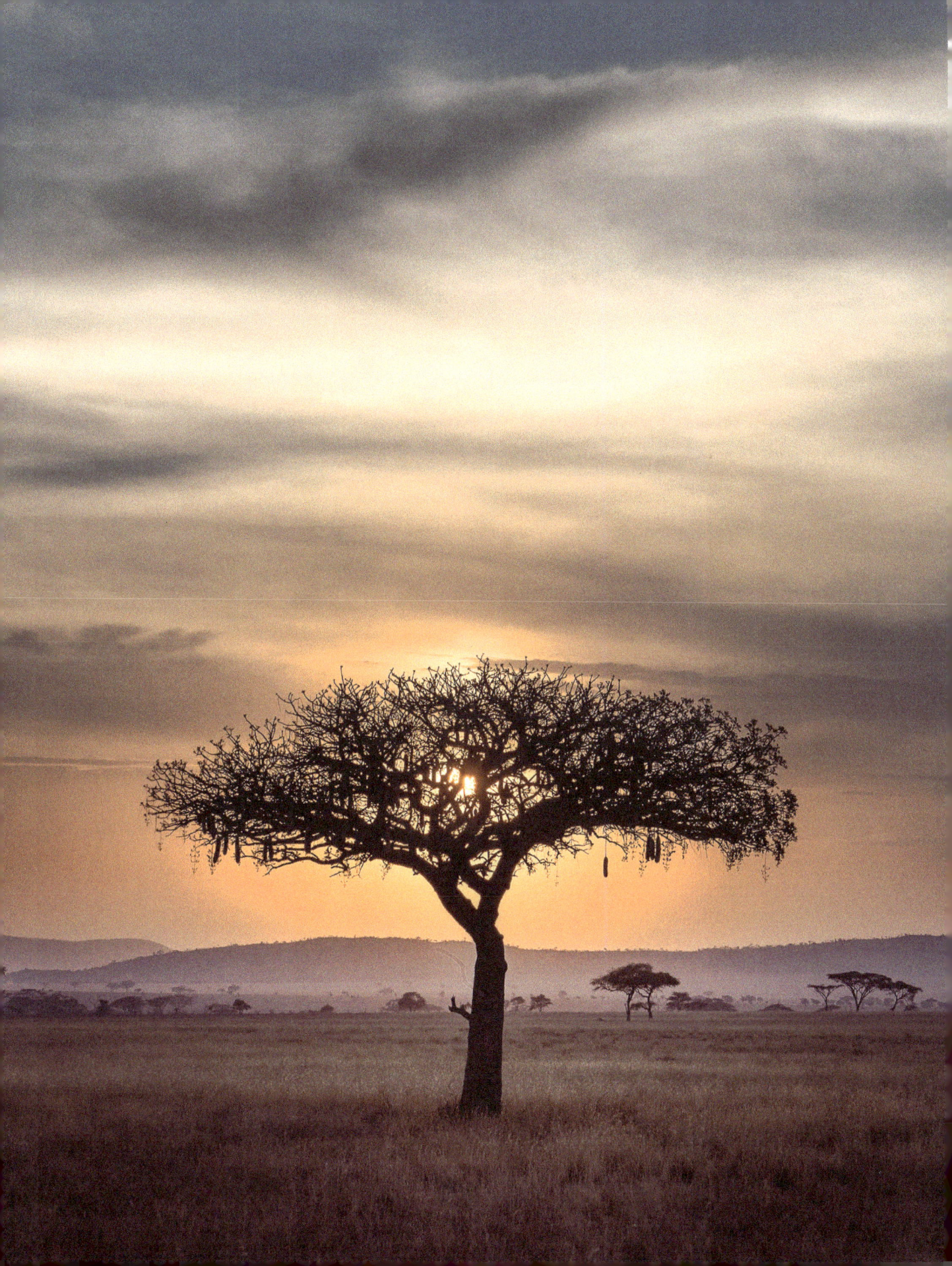

AFRIKAN YOGA?

The word 'yoga' is derived from the Sanskrit root 'yuj', which means 'union', 'join', or 'bring together'. It is taken from the Egyptian word 'Smai', which means 'union'.

This union is symbolic of the divine principle within and without us, our higher or real self. Yoga in the English word is 'yoke' and in the Latin is 'yugum', which when translated back to the English is 'married'. Now, Sanskrit is an Indo-Aryan language that was not spoken by the original inhabitants of India, known as Indus Kush in ancient times. Sanskrit was introduced to India around 1,500 B.C.

Smai has been practiced in Egypt, North Africa since at least 5,000 B.C, and earlier in the greater part of Egypt, Sudan, Ethiopia and Uganda. It was practiced by the Waab (priests), known in later times as Hery Heb (Teachers), and Sema (Funerary Priests) of Ancient Egypt, which is seen as hieroglyphs, reliefs, and statues dating thousands of years, showing the practices associated with yoga also existed on the African continent.

The word 'Smai', 'sema', or 'sem' is an Ancient Egyptian word meaning 'science of breath'. The Smai hieroglyph is commonly seen as a tube descending into a bulbous figure at the end of it.

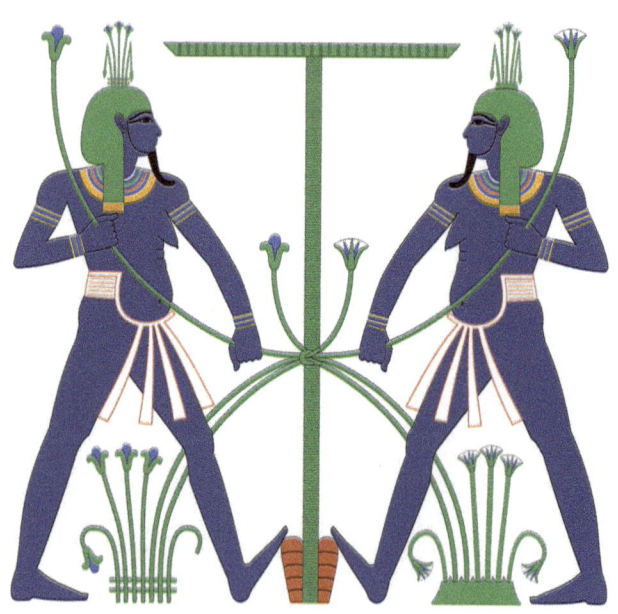

Taken from the relief found on the statue of Ramesses at Luxor Temple.

In the picture above, Smai is the central column, which in the human body represents the trachea, commonly called the windpipe, which descends down into the lungs. Its other meaning is the djed column or spine in the body with the pelvis attached to the end of the spine, as shown above, where the two figures of Hapi principle force of the Nile have their left and right feet on.

15 | THE RE-EMERGENCE OF TAMA-RE SMAI TAUI AFRIKAN YOGA

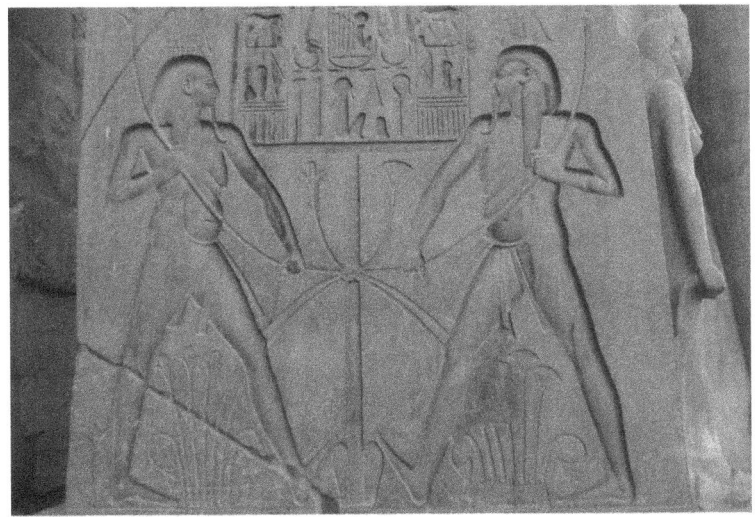

'Taui', 'tawi', or 'tawy' is the Ancient Egyptian word for two states which has been referred to as two lands, upper and lower Egypt. The two figures on either side, and the lotus and papyrus plants on either side representing the two lands. These lands or states have a multitude of meanings, internal and external, upper and lower natures, the self and the ego-self, the spiritual and the physical, and more – all referring to what can be seen as opposing forces that are bound together in order to work in a complementary way.

Smai Tawi: The Union of the Two Lands

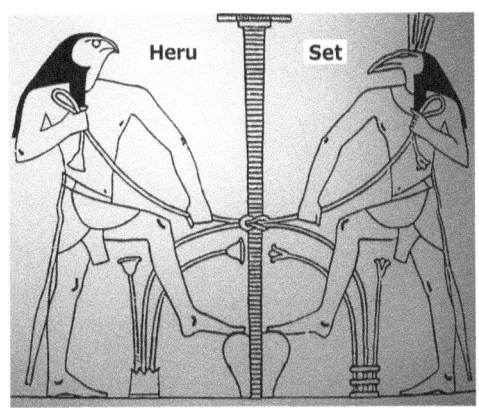

The two figures are seen on reliefs on temple walls and, at times, the two figures of Hapi interchange as Horus and Set tying the lotus and papyrus leaves together around the stem of the 'Nile', which represents the windpipe and spine of the body.

Smai Taui is the ancient health and wellbeing practice of Africa that can be called 'yoga' in India, 'Shin-Shin toitsu-do' in Japan, and 'Tai Chi' in China.

There are very few practitioners today who practise and at best teach this ancient healing art form from Africa.

> "As a rule, Egypt is always treated differently from the rest of the world. No Egyptologist has ever dreamed that the Ritual still exists under the disguise of both the gnostic and canonical gospels, [yogic philosophy and practices] or that it was the fountain-head and source of all the books of wisdom claimed to be divine."

Gerald Massey, *Egyptian Book of the Dead and the Mysteries of Amenta*

The various schools of Yoga include:

Hatha (Het Heru), the best-known school in the west, mainly, but not exclusively, physical.

Raja (Ra Ya) Yoga claims to be the highest yoga (Raja means 'royal') but omits the physical. This yoga is used intermittingly with Ashtanga yoga, another but more physical form of Hatha Yoga, and derived from the Indian Brahmin, Sri K. Pattabhi Jois.

Mantra (Ma NTR Ra) Japa and Nad Yoga concentrate on sound and meaning.

Swara (Shu Ra) Yoga concentrates on breathing.

Bhakti (Ba Akh Ta) Yoga's objectives are placed on devotional prayer, meditation, and selfless love.

Karma (Ka R Ma) Yoga concentrates on work and service.

Kundalini (Anu/Ureaus) Yoga focuses on the raising of the serpent or sekhem energy to integrate oneself with the higher consciousness (ANU).

Tantric (Ta NTR Ikh or Ta Nut Re) Yoga attains enlightenment through the union and balance of male and female energies either in sexual intercourse (Red Tantra or the left-hand path), in non-sexual (White Tantra or the right-hand path), or in abstraction (Black Tantra Yoga where the practice is shamanic, which refers to energy sensitivity, earth energy and shape-shifting/alchemy).

Afrikan (A free Ka) Yoga/ Tama-re Smai contains all the above with concentration on ancestral linkage, using them as examples of self-study and Haru/Heru as an example of self-mastery. Afrikan Yoga's ultimate goal is transcendence, union with nature, higher consciousness and the 'Most High'.

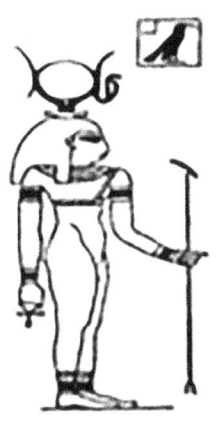

HATHA OR HAT HOR

Hatha is said to be two words combined: 'hat' sun and 'ha' moon. This meaning is not found in Sanskrit, must have had an older origin. The word 'Hatha' has a further root stemming back to Huwa, meaning 'creative force of will'.

In part, from the book *Solar Biology or Lunar Astrology* by Haru Hotep:

> "These eight elements were called Nu (Nawr), also called Nun (Nuwn) and Nunet (Naar); Heh (Huwa or Hatha) and Hehet (Hiya or Hathihi); Kek and Keket, the deities of darkness and void, who were responsible for removing the black dust cloud that covered the planet earth..."

Hatha derives from a principle or an action rather than a person and utilizes what is called 'the eight limbs':

1. **Yama** – non-violence, truthfulness, chastity, avoidance of greed.

2. **Niyama** – cleanliness of mind and body, devotion to God.

3. **Asanas** – the conditioning of the body through the postures to train the mind to achieve meditation (stillness and ultimate peace).

4. **Pranayama** – breath control and the utilization of sekhem to energize the body and relax the mind.

5. **Pratyahara** – teaches to withdraw the senses and not to overindulge in the external world.

6. **Dharana** – concentration on a subject for a short period of time. This is often developed through the use of asanas/postures.

7. **Dyama** – meditation which comes from a developed dharana (concentration).

8. **Samadhi** – deep meditation. This can be an outcome of all efforts combined to experience super/higher states of consciousness.

The modern-day styles that are born out of Hatha Classical Yoga are:

Ashtanga, Vinyasa, developed in Tibet and brought to the West by K. Pattabhi Jois.

Iyengar, whose study and emphasis is on alignment, developed in India and brought to the West by BKS Iyengar.

Power Yoga, developed in America by Beryl Bender Birch, with its emphasis on postures, the breath, heat, strength, and internalization – specific for American mentality.

Dynamic Yoga, developed in the UK by Godfrey Devereux (both dynamic yoga and power yoga are based on Ashtanga).

Bikram Yoga, 26 classical yoga postures performed in a heated room, developed in the USA by Bikram Choudhury.

I am often asked, "What is the difference between yoga (modern-day yoga) and Afrikan Yoga (Smai Tawi Ancient Tama-rean/Egyptian yoga)?" The Sanuyaat/postures seen in Afrikan yoga are numbered between 24 and 36, where modern-day yoga – that's what people mean when I am asked the difference – is now said to have 8,400 postures.

HATHA YOGA

Hatha yoga of 1000 ACE originally had very few postures, and it is not as ancient as many claim it to be. The elaborated movements seen today are certainly not ancient.

We are aware of Hatha as Huwa, creative force of will, and its foundations in Ancient Egypt (Afrika) as a science of intention and collaboration with the Neters through the use of breath and movement.

Het-Heru/.Hathor and Heru/Horus

Now for those of you who are aware of the meaning of the word 'Hatha', have you ever wondered why the pronunciation is Ha-fa instead of Hat (Sun) Ha (Moon)? Hatha is taken from Hathor, Het-Har or Het-Heru meaning 'the dwelling place of Heru'; the sacred cow deity of Ancient Egypt and also the consort of Heru. Hathor, the wife of Heru, gave birth to their son Har-smai tawy (Heru who unites the two lands). Hathor animal representation is the cow or heifer. The cow is well documented as the sacred animal of India and is worshipped as the symbol of a primordial mother.

In the Egyptian Prt M Heru, she is the one who urges the initiate to do battle with the monster Apep/Apophis. Apep in the mystical traditions is represented as the symbol of egoism that promotes thoughts, actions, and evil; so as not to lose [his or her] heart, she cries out, "Take your armour!" In a separate papyrus, the initiate is told that she (Het-Heru) is the one "who will make your face perfect among the Neters and Neterts, she will open your eye so that you may see every day... she will make your legs able to walk with ease in the Netherworld, Her name is Het-Heru, Lady of Amenta." Het-Heru/Hathor represents beauty, joyousness, love, and the bringer of happiness. Hathor is The Netert of the moon, the sky and the sun. A Netert of childbirth and young women, she is honoured as a mother and is synonymous with Aset; they are often associated with each other and share the same attributes. Het-Heru represents the power of Re, the supreme spirit, therefore associating with her implies coming into contact with the boundless source of energy that sustains the universe. She is the joyful, happy side of

Sakhmet, the fierce lioness who as the eye of Re, was an instrument of a destructive force and as the myth[1] goes began to slay men on earth to the point she got carried away and had to be subdued through the introduction of wine. Many European writers place emphasis on the wine aspect of the story, however, what is often missing in their writings is that Sakhmet as Hathor used dance, movement, and hikau (song), creative force that brought cheerfulness and raised the heavy spirit. This is the saving of mankind. Hathor/Hatha uses the elements of movement, posture, hikau, and a positive mentality to subdue the destructive forces of the ego. Het-Heru/Hathor imbues potency and healing and there are still dances and rituals in honour of her in the Sudan today, known as the 'Sacred cow dances'. Contact with Het-Heru implies developing inner will power and vitality, which engenders clarity of vision that will lead to the discovery of what is righteous and unrighteous (The practice of Afrikan Yoga/Tama-Re Smai Taui).

"Like everything else, life began with one thing in mind: to be, and with this thought a thing became, and impregnation existed by the will of Huhi as Hu (the creative force of will), who gave rule of this side of the universe to Re, making him the highest order of Sem."

Sacred Records of Atum Re 1:205

Yoga today, which derived from Smai, can be used as a means of reconnecting present-day Afrikans and people of the world to our higher selves (for Afrikans it is the Neter/Orisha/Annunagi) within and without. Smai/Yoga can be used to subdue the present destructive force within ourselves and our communities. This tool has lost its way through its Sanskrit meaning and now in the West has become quite beneficial, yet, of course, like all A Free Ka (n) Afrikan origins, through assimilation has lost its essence, its soul. The Sanuyaat postures explored in this book are on the walls in Ancient Egypt. The various 'Hanuaat' movements of The Neteru and Pharaohs are here for us to switch on our Hui/Hu creative force of will and transform again into Neters.

The All is I am

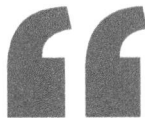

I am the Universe and the Universe is I
I am balanced, graceful and beautiful.
The Universe is balanced, graceful and beautiful.
I am the Universe and the Universe is I.

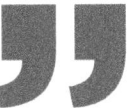

Khonsu Sekhem Ptah

---

[1] Wine is merely symbolic of the intoxicating feeling of the oneness with the supreme through 'the creative force of will' Hu.

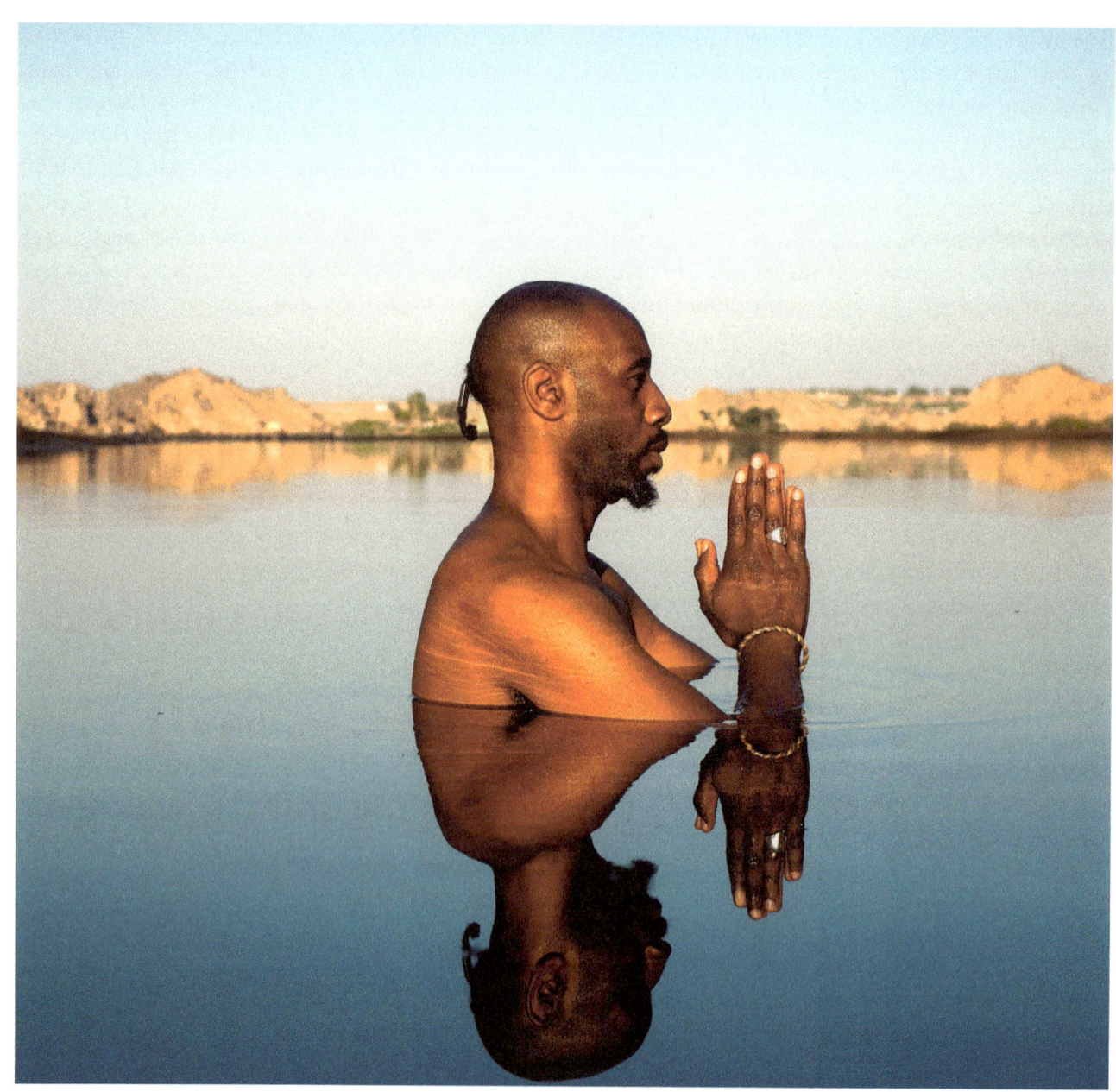

The Foundations
of Afrikan Yoga

Firstly, we have to deal with the word **'Ta'** in Tama-re, a name many of us call our children, sometimes pronounced and spelt Tamara or Tamerri. Ta is earth and is the grounding foundation of the aspirant. Ta, earth, is the first stage of the practice of Tama-re Smai Sanuyaat (forms). This principle is implemented to keep your feet firmly on the ground while exploring the god-head of Re. Ptah, the ancient deity of Kemet, father of Ra/Re, is the being who through the manifestation of thought and tone set the motion of creation through HuHi.

Ptah used the sound Aum, used by the mystics and spiritual aspirants today to stimulate higher senses, visualization and healing. Ptah is the being known to be the deity of physical creation; the creator of matter.

Ptah is pronounced Tar. The earliest of the ancient names of Egypt is Tar ('Black as tar' comes to mind when speaking of the Tarites).

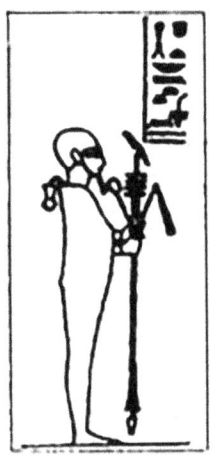

The 'Pygmy', or should I say an insulting name calling of the ancient peoples of Afrika, whose true name[2] is Ptahrites or Tarites, were your pre-history, pre-dynastic people of Ancient Khemet KMT, known as TA MA RE, who were indigenous to the planet. They studied how to manipulate the elements through the mind, soul, and spirit. They were remembered and deified just as Michael Jordon, Pele, Muhammad Ali, or Billie Holiday are honoured today. The elements and principles began to have a face and name in remembrance of these great masters and, in turn, we found inspiration and a connection through a blood-link, a genetic re-coding, which on further inspection leads into atoms, back to the un-manifested, back to the source. This is one of our many tools of connectivity.

The deity Ptah, whose wife was Sekhmet and his son Neferten (or Nefertem/Nefertum), made up the Memphite triad or Trinity.

Ptah was associated with Hephasteus by the Greeks. He was the deity of blacksmiths; the Romans called him Vulcan after their own God of the forge.

Ptah invented the methods and techniques of the craftsmen and was the deity of masons; his high priests held the title 'Master Builder' or 'Supreme Leader of Craftsmen'. This forging done by the original blacksmiths was the forging of the internal and the eternal soul, the transformational development of one's character.

The Ptarhites were small people, about 4ft

---

[2] **Note:** However, throughout time we are known and called by many names and what you choose to call yourself must have a connection to your culture, land, dress, customs and laws that ultimately reflect all the above. Black by modern day definition has no culture, etc., and appears to be just a colour: this, too, is an illusion.

tall, yet they were mental giants.

Note: Ptah was an earth deity and had links with the underworld.

Secondly, the word '**Ma**' derives from Tama-rean Nuwaupic and the metu neter word 'ma' or 'mu' for water, and it is also the first two letters in Ma'at.

Ma'at is the ancient one who represents the symbol of truth, justice and world order, and is the female deity of weighing the Ab 'heart'. Ma'at always wears the ostrich feather, a symbol of law, truth, right, and justice. The word Ma'at means 'that which is straight, right, true, sincere, and honest' and perhaps even 'Tao' or 'balance'. She is the woman of the judgement hall; her feather was balanced against the heart of the deceased to determine whether he had led a pure and honest life. Ma'at was represented as a tall woman with an ostrich feather in her hair. Ma'at is the wife of Tehuti, Djehuti, Zehuti (Thoth), and the Daughter of Re. She assisted Ptah (pronounced Tar) and Khnum in carrying out rightly the work of creation order by Tehuti. She is the order that rules the world through balance.

Ma'at's symbol, the ostrich feather, is also the quill and the hand symbol Yod, or Y which is the letter I (I and Y are interchangeable in the old languages), as in I in Egipt. I is the 9th letter of the alphabet and 9 is the highest number, 9 to 9th power, nine mind, etc. The use of the hand was adopted by the monotheists and became the hand of God, Allah or Jehovah. The ostrich feather was used as a pen for writing the hieratic script of Ta-Mara, Tama-re. The feather is interchangeable with the beak of the Ibis bird for the deity Tehuti which symbolised the scribe that wrote the law of the Torah and the Bible. This, in turn, gave birth to the Qu'ran (Koran), all taken from the Egiptians, when the God of the Torah Yahweh was supposed to have written it by hand for the Haribu-aat (Hebrews). The Rabbis show the symbol of the extended finger, which originally came from the beak of the Ibis bird, under Mose, who became Moses, Mosheh (Judaism) and Muwsa (Islamism). All from the Egiptian Mose meaning 'child' of the school of Thothmose, who was a student of Thoth. Tehuti, who became Hermes, from the Latin Hermeticus, meaning 'alchemical' was borrowed by the Greeks and used as a god, son of Zeus and Maia.

In the words of The Master Teacher Amunnubi Ruakh Ptah, **"Ma'at is the pillar of justice and is the spiritual struggle against injustice. We, the Tama-reans, must learn to assimilate, to distribute and to pass judgment justly and with impartiality. We must stand for true Ma'at, 'that which is right'."**

The declarations of Ma'at known as the 42 declarations of innocence are the principal basis of the Ten Commandments.

By a conservative estimate, the 42 Oracular Principles of Ma'at (Declarations of Innocence) were written approximately 1,500 years before the writing of the Ten Commandments. By comparing the two documents, one will find striking similarities. The 42 Oracular Principles of Ma'at are drawn from the A Free Ka (n) Holy book Prt m Hru (*Book of Coming Forth by Day*), the world's oldest book of Holy scriptures. With these laws, our ancient ancestors maintained a society without a police force for thousands of years. In the early morning say, "I will not", and in the evening say, "I have not..." This is how we perform a moral inventory.

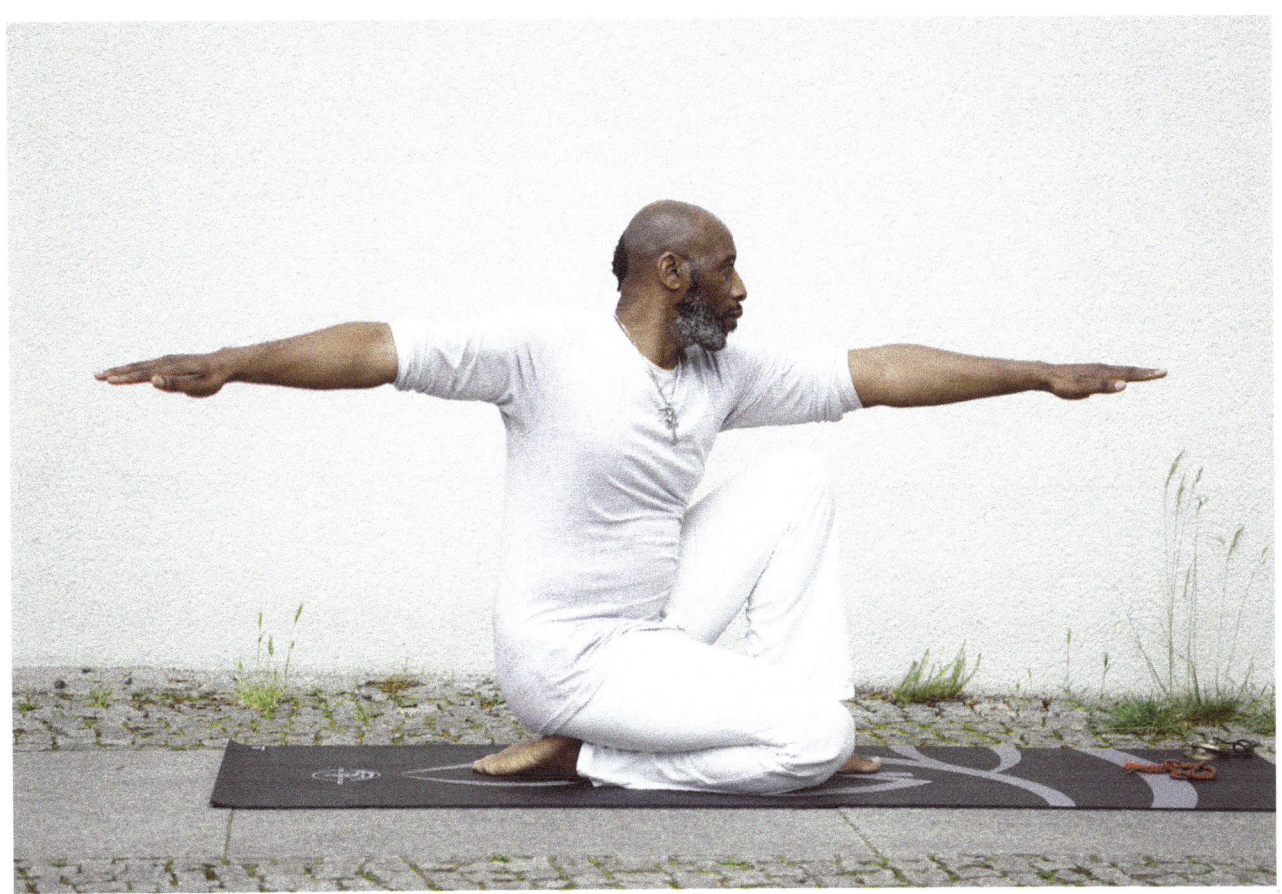

NETERT MA'AT

THE 42 ORACULAR PRINCIPLES OF Ma'at
(PRT M HRU)

Translation by Pablo M Imani

For the morning declare:

1. I **Will Not** do wrong
2. I **Will Not** steal, rob, cheat
3. I **Will Not** act with violence (brutalize)
4. I **Will Not** kill (cause murder for sport)
5. I **Will Not** be unjust (biased)
6. I **Will Not** cause pain (inflict cruelty, torture, or needless injury)
7. I **Will Not** waste food or squander resources
8. I **Will Not** lie (perjure)
9. I **Will Not** desecrate holy places (be irreverent)
10. I **Will Not** speak evil
11. I **Will Not** abuse my sexuality
12. I **Will Not** cause the shedding of tears
13. I **Will Not** sow seeds of regret

14. I **Will Not** be an aggressor
15. I **Will Not** act guilefully
16. I **Will Not** lay waste to the land
17. I **Will Not** bear false witness
18. I **Will Not** set my mouth in motion against any person
19. I **Will Not** be wrathful or angry except for a just cause
20. I **Will Not** copulate with a man's wife or a woman's husband
21. I **Will Not** desecrate the wife of a man or husband of a woman (commit adultery)
22. I **Will Not** pollute myself (my body temple)
23. I **Will Not** cause terror
24. I **Will Not** pollute the earth
25. I **Will Not** speak in anger
26. I **Will Not** turn from the words of right and truth (disobedience to one's conscience)
27. I **Will Not** utter curses (debase my power of speech)
28. I **Will Not** initiate a quarrel (instigate disharmony)
29. I **Will Not** be excitable or contentious (impatient)
30. I **Will Not** prejudge (be presumptuous)
31. I **Will Not** be an eavesdropper
32. I **Will Not** speak over much
33. I **Will Not** commit treason against the ancestors
34. I **Will Not** waste water
35. I **Will Not** do evil
36. I **Will Not** be arrogant (insolent)
37. I **Will Not** blaspheme NTR (The Highest Mother-Father of Creation)
38. I **Will Not** commit fraud
39. I **Will Not** defraud Temple offerings
40. I **Will Not** plunder the dead (grave robbery, piracy)
41. I **Will Not** mistreat/abuse children
42. I **Will Not** mistreat/abuse animals

Repeat in the evening and declare, "I have not…"

The ten virtues of the initiates under the guidance of Ma'at and Tehuti

Afrikan Yogic Philosophy:

1. Control your thoughts
2. Control your actions
3. Have devotion and purpose
4. Have faith in your master's ability to lead you along the path of truth
5. Have faith in your own ability to accept the truth
6. Have faith in your ability to act with wisdom
7. Be free from resentment under the experience of persecution

8. Be free from resentment under the experience of wrong

9. Learn and know how to distinguish right and wrong

10. Learn and know how to distinguish the real from the unreal

Adorations to Ma'at

(Berlin Papyrus) Afrikan Yogic Philosophy
Ma'at Ankhu Ma'at – Ma'at is the source of life

Ma'at Neb Buten – Ma'at is in everywhere you are
Kha Hena Ma'at – Rise in the morning with Ma'at
Ankh Hena Ma'at – Live with Ma'at
Ha Senna Ma'at – Let every limb join with Ma'at
Ma'at Her Ten – Ma'at is who you are deep down
Dua Ma'at Neb Buten – Adorations/Thanks to Ma'at who is everywhere you are

Hymn to Ma'at in the Temple of Amun El Hibis, translation by Pablo M Imani

Praise to you, Ma'at, daughter of Ra, consort of NTR, whom Ptah loves, the one who adorns the breast of Tehuti, who formed her own nature, foremost of the souls of Annu;

Who pacified the two falcons NTRU through her goodwill, filled the Per-Wer shrine (Great House) with life and dominion;

The skilled one who brought forth the NTRU herself and brought low the heads of enemies;

Who herself provides for the house of Nebertcher;

She brings daily offerings for those who are on duty;

Magnificent her throne before the judges and she consumes the enemies of Atum/Anu

Ma

The principle of water is of a feminine nature and utilises patience, perseverance and creative energies in order to grow and nurture seeds. We may only look at a few ancestral deities of water to clearly understand water principles.

The deity Tefnut is moisture and is represented in the *'Hanuaat'* movements, *'Hudu'* Afrikan Tai Chi and *'Ragus'* dance of Afrikan Yoga/Tama-re Smai Taui.

"The word Ma is water, which symbolises the womb, or the embryonic sac that the foetus rests in before leaving the womb, it's the primordial water."

Sacred Records of Atum Re (scroll 1.129)

The Afrikan cosmology of the 8 Rashunaat also known as the Khemenu (8), Ogdoads

These beings are known as the primordial ancestors or the Adams and Eves, also known to form the primary creative and cosmic 8 forces of the womb of existence known as Nun, which means potential and our boundless universe, related to the Odu in Ifa and the I ching. The Khemenu, Ogdoads deal with time and space, the cardinal points, the two solstices, the two equinoxes, and the four midpoints commonly referred to as the four seasons. The Khemenu, Ogdoads came also to represent periods of time in our evolution and are often noted by European writers as tadpoles, reptilians, and frogs: this is why the word evolution is apt as they are the symbolic development of growth throughout time and also within the womb of our mother. Ever wondered why in our English schools they made you do experiments on frogs in biology class? This is because a frog laid out is close to the human anatomy.

The first set: Nun / Nunet

Neter Nun   Netert Nunet

They are the first stage of our evolved state; the sea-men and the first period of gestation. Nun is the male part meaning 'deep abyss', 'chaos', and Nunet is the female consort meaning 'the abyss'. They are the deities of water. A third of the human body is water, and the lymphatic and circulatory systems are the source of life and reproduction. Water is the most important element in existence and a needed source of conduction.

The second set: Heh / Hehet

Neter Heh   Netert Hehet

The second set of our evolution is represented by the male Neter Heh 'infinity' and his female consort Netert Hehet 'eternity'. They were also known as the deities of immeasurable time and were represented by tadpoles.

The third set: Khek / Kheket

Neter Khek   Netert Kheket

The third state of our evolution is Neter Khek, the male deity of supreme darkness, and Netert Kheket, the female deity of Supreme darkness.

The fourth set: Amun / Amunet

Neter Amun   Netert Amunet

Amun, 'the hidden one', is the male part and Amunet, 'she who is hidden', the female consort. They are the deities that bred on earth and are the earth deities or our very first Adams and Eves, human beings who breathed.

The first three were your original water beings and show our basic stages of evolution that are played out through nine months of pregnancy. That follows our watery beginnings into breathing Adams coming out of the darkness of the womb. Our Ancient Afrikan scientists are well aware of this and symbolised them through our many stories of creation.

Maybe we should rename this planet H_2O because it has far more water on it than earth and all the water is connected, from the rivers to the streams, to the oceans, to even the clouds. The continents sit on top of the water and have been drifting since the pre-Cambrian age. This is an aquarium for there is water in the air and absolutely everything else on this planet. From your rocks to your plastics, which will somehow contain water, and our bodies are made up of over 70 per cent of the substance: we would absolutely shrivel and die without it. Our skins would peel and flake like that of reptiles' if we did not submerge ourselves in water every day.

Water is fundamental and we need to take it to keep ourselves in a state of good health and, of course, social inclusion.

Drew Fobbester, an online nutritionist, says, "If you want well-moisturized skin, hydrate. If you did nothing else but drink at least eight glasses a day, you would see a huge improvement in your skin." NO amount of Oil of Olay will moisturize your skin like water and nourishing food do, which may prove to be a better investment in having and maintaining lustrous skin and glowing health.

Truth is, we are water beings; from the sperm seaman/semen to the egg, we function in water.

RE

The word 'Re' or tone Ray in Tama-re is the final principle in our school. This tone brings together all other tones and is a key element in all things.

For example:

Music: Do Ray Mi Fa Sol La (solar) Te Do

Science: Resonance, Regeneration, Relativity, Resolution, Response, Respiration

Art: Re-creation

Mathematics: Reciprocal, Reflection, Reflex, Rectangle, and Revolution

Re align, Re member, Re spect, Re turn: this is an oscillation, a vibratory rate of creation, bringing something, anything, into existence, and this creation is constant like thoughts. Re is to do again, and again, and again. That is why it is a prefix word and sound in every repeated action in the Dictionary (definitionary), and if any form of creation is hidden, it will eventually be exposed, again and again by the physical or spiritual sun. This being is one we must acquaint ourselves with as this is the Most High being. Supreme Being of supreme beings, Ra is actually Greek and is the later form of Re (Ray) of Ancient Egypt. Re was the name given to the sun by the Egyptians. RE is the sun or solar deity, the fire principle dealing with heat, light, vitality, knowledge, and creation.

The physical sun of our solar system is symbolic as it is the firstborn, giving birth to our planets and is so vital to our lives, that if the sun was blocked out for an entire day, everything on this planet would begin to die.

The sun is about 93 million miles away, its temperature on the surface is around 9,980F and at its core, the temperature is approx. 27,000,0000F – this is to say that the Ancient Afrikans are spot on when they relate themselves and all things in creation to the number 9. RE origins were in the water of Nun, having his eyes and mouth shut. After becoming tired of his inactivity, he climbed from the darkness, showing himself in all his glory. RE predates Allah, whose plural is Allahumma (Quran 5 times 3:26, 3:17, 8:32, 10:10, 39:36): the word means 'Oh, Allah, the source'. Allahumma is another word that was derived from the Hebrew word Eloheem, found in the Torah 430 times, meaning 'these beings' or *'a group of Elohs, the Gods'*. The attributes of Allah coincide with the 99 elements, which can be traced further back to the 99 ancient ancestors or Neters, which I will show further in this book. The 36th Attribute of Allah, called Al Aliyu, 'The Most High', is also the name of the 86th chapter of the

Koran today, which was originally called Suwrah Al Ala, 'Chapter of the Most High'. Muslims use the 36th attribute of Allah Al Aliyu, 'The Most High', when they say, 'Allahu Subhanna Wa Ta' Ala', Glory be to Allah the Most High, or in short 'Allah Ta'Ala', Alla the Most High, as in Genesis 14:18 and Koran 87:1. 'The Most High God' in Hebrew is Elyuwn Elyuwn El. It can be found in the Bible a total of 43 times.

The 93rd Attribute of Allah is 'Al Nuwr', The Light (Koran 24:35), 'The source, Allah is the Nuwr, light of the samawati, skies and the planet earth'. RE, the visible emblem of the Most High ANU, was regarded as the head of the YAHWEH, meaning, 'He who is, who he is' or the NETERU, NETERS, nature, the personification of the 99 elements, the Elders, Ancestors. Re has many forms. One that was the most important was the one where he is seen with a falcon head wearing a Solar Disk and Ureas.

PA RE the sun is the source of life and without this source, I repeat, all on this planet would die as the ecosystems of the earth are sustained by Re. Our ancients recognised this crucial source and were seen to be sun worshippers. This is but a misinterpretation on the part of those who robbed the graves, tombs and temples of Ancient Khemet. The actual source of sun worship was originally the sun inside, not the sun outside, but in reference to the solar plexus, our central system, and second brain, also known as central intelligence. As was taught by The Supreme Spiritual Master Amunnubi Ruakh Ptah, *"Re symbolises Universal Consciousness, and in man individual consciousness. Consciousness is the receiving capacity of the soul or individual intelligence."*

The Solar plexus sits within the centre of our digestive system, the carrier of our emotions. The digestion begins at the mouth and ends at the rectum. The Solar plexus is also depicted with the colour yellow which is the colour of intellect.

RE is attributed as the all-seeing eye, of which all the occultists are aware, yet by many has been taught as the evil eye which has misinformed many. This All Seeing Eye comes from the ability to be present and consciously aware. To be present and not seen is the skill of invisibility, which leads to **Amun**. Amun is the hidden principle of Re and Re is the personification of Amun. Amun, who is also called Amen, Amin, Ameen, Iman, Imani, and Mu'min, is still being worshipped today by Jews, Christians and Muslims; all their prayers end with Amen meaning *'faith'*.

These principles are the foundation and make up you, the *Smai Afrikan Yogi*, who is the worker of *'Nine Mind'*.

The mutalub/student of Smai is well aware of these principles; they are well aware of the principle forces of nature/guardians that govern them and strive to grasp the inner workings of the cosmology pertaining to his/herself, also known as the inner mysteries as well as the outer mysteries. This is the very thing that they teach. This is the essential behind the symbology. They progress further as they are now rooted in the Nine. The Smai practitioner utilises the 'Science of Nine Ether', which in essence is a series of principles. It is evident that these principles have to some become more of a religion. Religions breed hatred, separation, racism, ignorance, and war as the ego is an entity that feels disconnected from All. The ego perceives itself constantly under threat and seeks out constant conflict within and without. Within religions, the personalities (Jesus, Buddha, Muhammad, Moses) take over the teachings, giving birth to further personalities (Pastors, Missionaries, Monks, Rabbis, and Imams), staunch followers, and egotistic entities, who strip the higher teachings down into a series of dos and don'ts, good and bad, a series of polarities and dichotomies.

As human beings, we struggle with these parameters and will keep struggling with them constantly for these lower mysteries do not allow for GOD consciousness to truly prevail as they do not enhance our divinity – they eventually become a matrix. Like all religions, when stripped down to their bare essentials, the underlining principles lead one to a higher state of consciousness. Hru (God Consciousness) can in no way be mentally understood and there is no intellectual agreement. Hru (God Consciousness) must be felt completely with every cell of your body and every connection of your being. Hru (God Consciousness) is unspoken, unwritten, the un-manifested. The time is truly now, when you, The Afrikan, must realise the science you prescribe to cannot be found outside of yourself in any church, synagogue, temple, tabernacle. It can only be found waiting in silence within, where the truth of you, your wants, your wishes and the universe moves as one flow, like a stream of universal beauty. There within is your power and your connection with your divine self. The practice of Afrikan Yoga 'Smai' is a key component in my realisation of this fact as I used movement, body awareness, breath, and meditation (inner stillness) to facilitate a higher consciousness: a journey where emotions and ego are watched all the way; a journey where intensity, presence and living are evenly matched in a pool of timelessness, no-thing and no separation.

It is a journey we really call transformation, as the ancient alchemists spoke of concerning the change from base metals into gold; where you shine like the sun and no negativity can reside in you, and no negativity can sit beside you and not be transformed.

"I am the Great One, the son of a Great One. I am the Fiery One, the son of a Fiery One, whose head was restored to him after it had been cut off. The head of Osiris, the Risen Saviour, is not taken from him and my head shall not be taken from me. I have risen up and knitted myself together. I have made myself whole. I renew myself and grow young again. I am one with Osiris, Lord of Eternity."

The Book of Coming Forth by Day, **Atum**

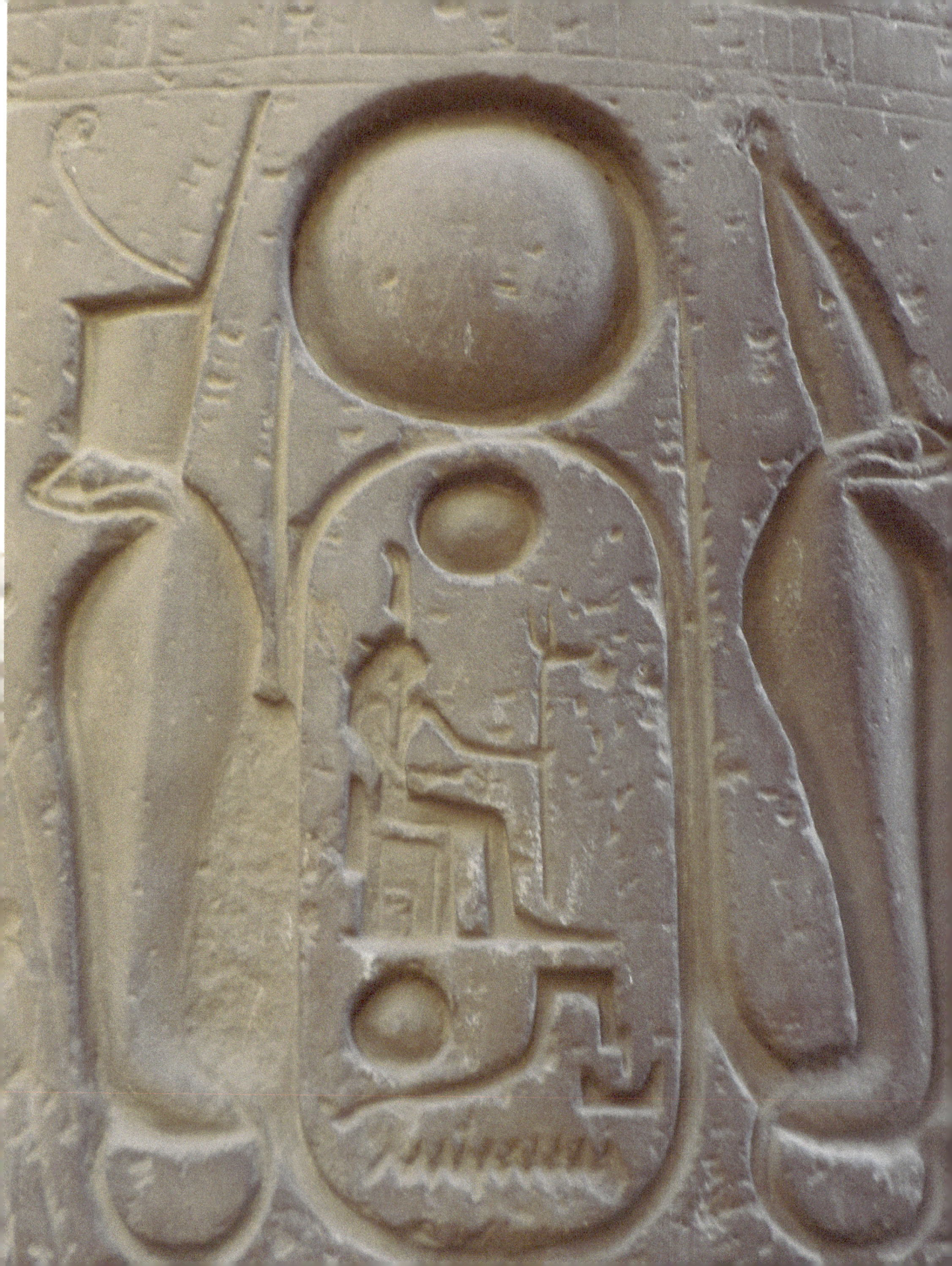

THE RADIANCE OF A GREAT MASTER TEACHER'S TOOL

> "The greatest challenge for the initiate is to refrain from taking sides in the seeming conflicts of life. All adversities exist for the sake of making demands upon the individual to reach into the depths of his/her spirit to awaken the spiritual power to overcome them. One cannot push, exert force if there is no opposition, there can be no manifestation of spiritual power without adversity. All is peace. Hetep."

Ra Un Nefer Amen, Medu Neter Vol 1.

I know this to be true seeing the countless obstacles in life I have personally encountered as a means to my growth, and seeing the many conflicts family and friends have suffered to a bitter end or to overwhelming joy and expansion of their lives. The master tool in the recognition of such onslaughts on one's hetep/peace is the wisdom of Tehuti, an invaluable resource for understanding the laws of mind. However, these laws are themselves illusions, a matrix of which we must rise above or delve deeper into being in order to be one, to reconnect to our true self: the self-connected to all things. They must be overstood.

Before speaking about TEHUTI and the principles also known as laws, let me relay an experience that gave me a deeper insight into this master.

While practising Vipassana Meditation under the guidance of S.N Goenka, a teacher of Indian descent born in Burma and devout Buddhist, also a teacher of thousands of people in more than 350 courses in India and other countries, East and West, who had become a master of Meditation, I received what is known as internal insight. The technique, which S.N Goenka teaches, represents a tradition that is traced back to the Buddha. In short, the technique is one of self-observation that shows reality in its two aspects, inner and outer. In the language of India at the time of Buddha, passana meant to look, to see things in an ordinary way; vipassana is to observe things as they really are, not just as they seem to be. Apparent truth had to be penetrated until one reached the ultimate truth of the entire mental and physical structure.

During this time a question kept on rearing its head, "Who is Buddha?"

Strict observations of silence, called 'Noble Silence' for nine days, 10 hrs of meditation a day, had to be adhered to for 10 days (courses can last up to 30 days). In the first two days, when permitted, I began to ask the assistant teachers about Buddha. Of course, short and brief answers were returned. Gautama Buddha was not the first; there were many Buddhas and Gautama was part of a spiritual lineage. Listening to the discourses of S.N Goenka, the axioms he used from the teachings of Buddha resembled the **Hah Kha,** the sacred wisdom teachings of Tehuti, also known as the greater mysteries which gave birth to the lesser mysteries: Christianity, Judaism, and Islam. I found myself in the wisdom school, the school of Tehuti *naturally*. The **Hah Kha** resurfaced today by the Spiritual Master teacher, Amunnubi Ruakh Ptah. I was able to recognize all the axioms presented and this intensified my question, "So who was the first Buddha?" In exploring my structure day after day during meditation the answer sparked; the answer was, "Buddha, who gave birth to a line of spiritual aspirants, was no other than The Grand Hierophant Tehuti himself." Gautama Buddha was a student of Dravidian yogis as well as Tehuti. Gautama proved the maxims of the original teachings for himself by sitting for long periods of time in meditation. "Be still and know that I Am God." This speaks of the God within, the divine self and instructs an awakening to pure consciousness devoid of attachments and the ramblings of the mind. Tehuti, or in Greek, Thoth (where we get the word 'thought' from), derived certain principles, maxims and axioms to assist the realization of true consciousness. Buddha means the 'awakened one'. This literally means that you can be Buddha as and when you awaken in your own lifetime, today, and not some distant future, and is not just an exclusive experience of Siddhartha Gautama as the Buddhists believe.

Note: I recommend that all Smai/yoga aspirants take up this practice and perform nine days of noble silence with 10 full hours of Meditation daily once a year to maintain and develop their inner wisdom. I'll explain my reasoning behind this by adding the comments of Dr Muata Ashby from his book *African Origins of Civilization, Religion and Yoga Spirituality*:

"The origins of Hatha Yoga were clearly in Buddhism and not in Hinduism since we find evidence of rejection of Hatha Yoga by the Hindu sages. Hatha Yoga is clearly rejected in the Laghu-Yoga – Vaisistha (5.6.86, 92), which maintains that it merely leads to pain; some of criticisms, especially against the magical undercurrents." Dr Muata Ashby continues further saying, *"Specifically, Tantric Buddhism gave rise to the earliest practice of certain postures as a means to enhance spiritual evolution. Before this time, the only reference to asana or posture was the sitting posture for meditation mentioned in the Raja Yoga Sutras by Pantanjali. STHIRA SUKHAM ASANAM. STHIRA: Steady. SUKHAM: Comfortable. ASANAM: Pose (for meditation). Meaning: A seated pose (for meditation) that is steady and comfortable is called Asana.*

"To attain success in the practice of concentration, meditation and Samadhi, an aspirant begins by developing steadiness of a meditative pose.

"Buddhist records show that early Buddhists had visited Memphis [Sakkara/Tattu, the Nome or city of Ptah – author's addition] and set up a settlement there. Henceforth Buddhism begins to develop similar iconographies including the Divinity sitting on the lotus, ... similar to those of Ancient Egypt..."

To encase this further: "In Ancient Kamit there were at least 24 postures in the spiritual practice prior to the time of Pantajali. In the practice of Kamitian Tjef Neteru (Egyptian Hatha Yoga), the 'magic' consists of using postures to engender certain alignments with spiritual energies and cosmic forces. This is the kind of practice repudiated by the Hindu sages and adopted by the Tantric Buddhists. Between the years 100 A.C.E. and 1000 A.C.E., the Buddhist Kaula School developed some postures. Then Goraksha developed what is regarded by present-day Hatha Yoga practitioners as a practice similar to the present day. However, the number of postures only reached 15 at the time of Hatha Yoga Pradipika scripture. The Mysore family was instrumental in the development since they were strong patrons of Hatha Yoga. Subsequent teachers developed more postures and vinyasa (which was not practised in early Indian Hatha Yoga) up to the 20th century where there are over 200. The teacher Krishnamacharya said he had learned from a yoga teacher in Tibet. Krishnamacharya's first writings, which cited the Stitattvandihi as a source, also featured vinyasa (sequences of poses synchronized with the breath) that Krishnamacharya said he had learned from a teacher in Tibet. So the practice of the postures in India does not extend to ancient times and did not begin in India with Hinduism but with Buddhism, and Buddhism was associated with the Ancient Egyptian city of Memphis where postures and spiritual magic were practised previously."

The father of 'magic' is Tehuti and in order to perform magic and not tricks, there is a great emphasis on mastering your thoughts and controlling your mind, which can only be achieved through meditation. The Greeks had translated the name Tehuti to Thoth, which when observed, seems innocent and just a transliteration. However, Thoth gives us the word thought, and it is thoughts that cause us to miss constantly the ultimate reality, pure joy, pure love, and freedom found in the state of 'NOW' only to oscillate between the past and future, good and bad, meaning being in a state of duality. That is why as descendants of these great masters and ancestors we cannot afford to lean too much on Greek translations of our ancient names and places. Return to the Great Master's tool meditation and regain the mastery of your mind; within this process, you have access to all the answers you need.

Buddha was Black, that's why his woolly hair is always shown in small tight curls, peppercorn style, or cornrows. Early sculptures of him clearly reveal his Africoid features... wide nose and full lips. So was Zaha of Japan, Fu-Hsi of China, Tyr of Scandinavia, Quetzalcoatl of Mexico, Sommonacom of Siam and Isis of Egypt and Rome. Krishna of India was 'blue-black'.

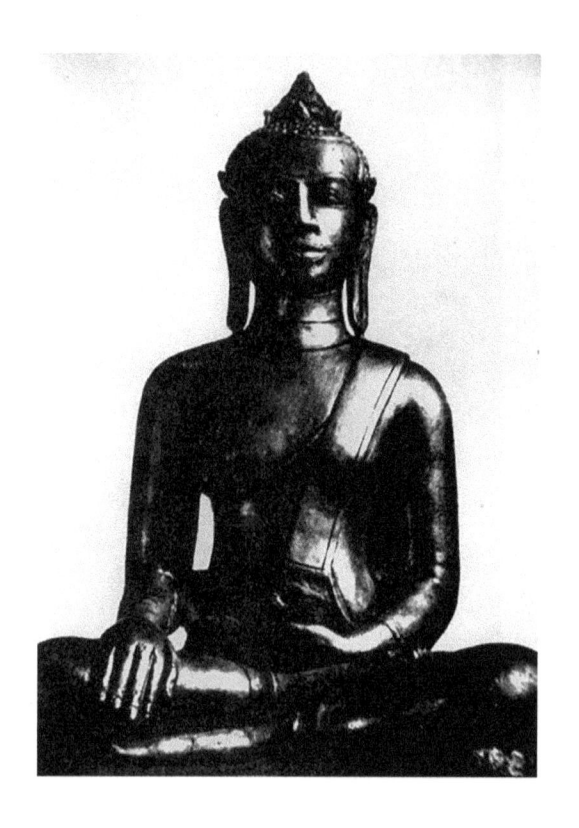

The historical Buddha was not the first, he had many predecessors. Tehuti was the first Buddha. One of his students, Zoser, built the step pyramid in Saqqara. He was also a Buddha and a High Priest of Tehuti. Tehuti was known in many cultures as:

Hermes Trismegistus (Greek)

Thoth (Greco-Egypt)
Mercury (Rome)

Quetzalcoatl (Mexico)

Rapanui (Easter Island)

Nabu/Nebu (Assyrian)

Abdul Quduws (Arabia)

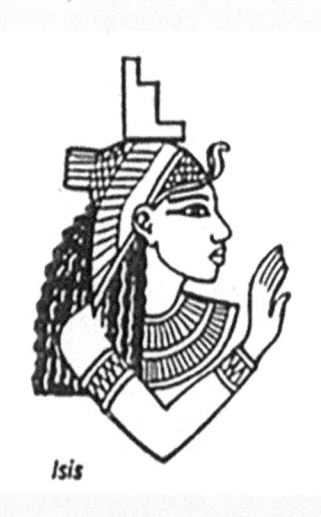

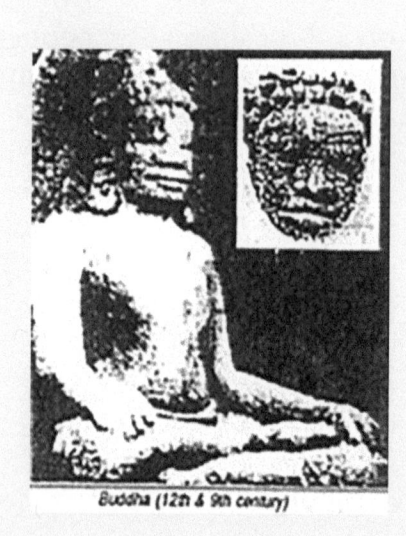

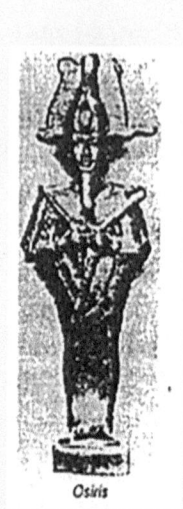

Isis

Buddha (12th & 9th century)

Osiris

These great sages cannot be denied and to say they were otherwise when drawn images and carved stones depict them Afrikan is to reveal a mental health and a pathological issue.

TEHUTI/DJEHUTI

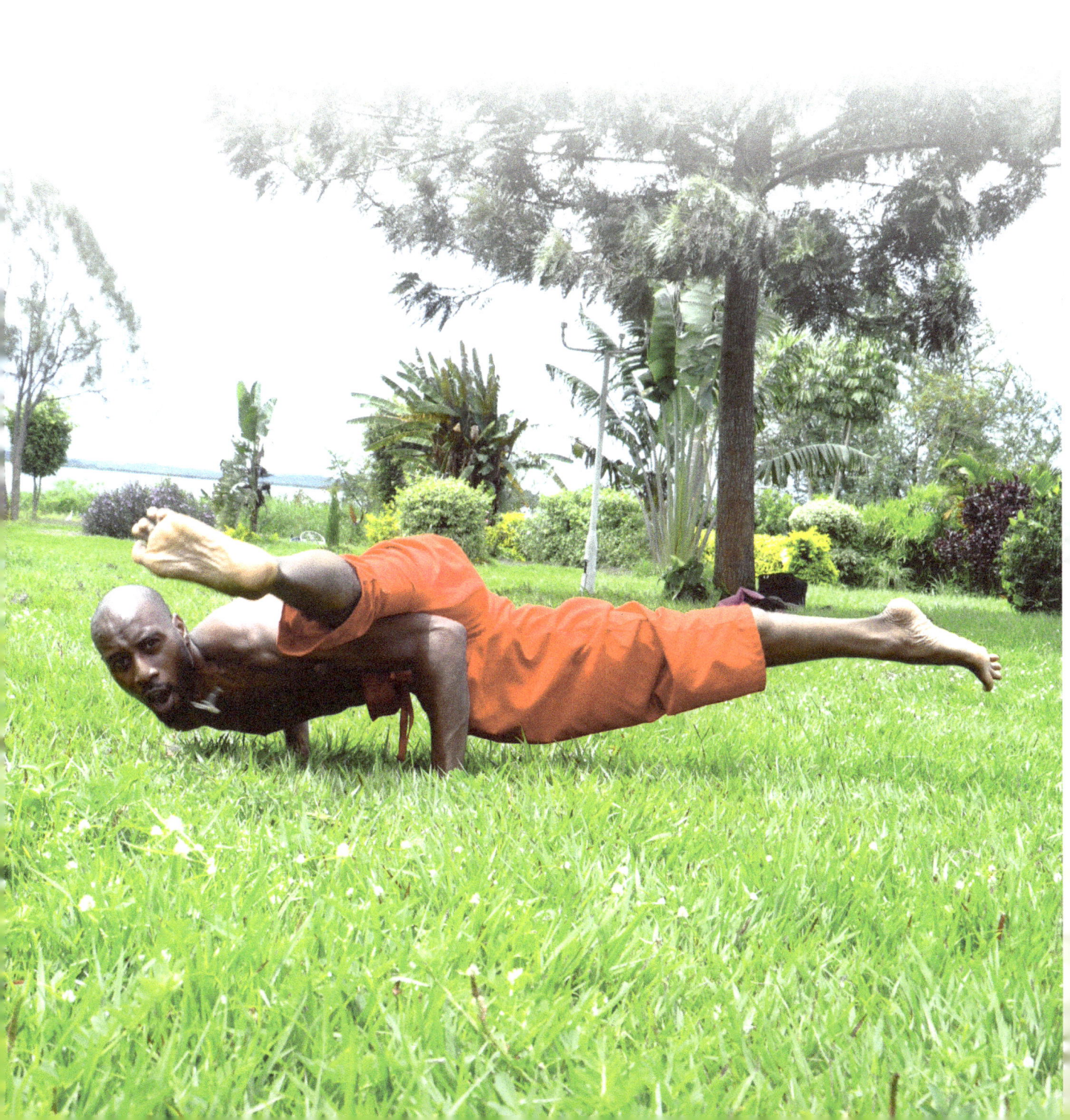

Named by the Greeks (the so-called foundation of European thought and culture), Thoth had many names: Tehuty, Dihuty, Dhouti, Thout, Zehuti, Sheps, and Lord of the Khemenu, Father Time.

Djehuty 'Leader' Ibis-headed Lord of Time, Writing, and Wisdom, Djehuty is a scribe who wrote the story of our reality.

The name Thoth means 'Truth' and 'Time'. Thoth was the Master architect who created the blueprint of our reality based on the mathematics of sacred geometry and placed it in Grids (A Matrix) for us to experience and learn.

It also has been said that he invented the hieroglyphic script and negotiated five extra days from the moon in order to perfect the 365-day year. As a result of these mythological connections, he is also known as the deity of the moon and the moon cycle. Djehuty is the patron of writers, teachers, accountants, and all persons involved in the dissemination of knowledge, writing, and/or calculation. His consorts are alternately **Ma'at,** Netert of Truth and Order, or Seshat, patroness of record-keeping, libraries and the foundation of buildings.

It was Tehuti who helped Aset work the ritual to bring Asaru back from the dead and who drove the magical poison of Set from her son, Haru, with the power of his magic. He was Haru's supporter during the young deity's deadly battle with his uncle Set, helping Haru with his wisdom and magic. It was Tehuti who brought Tefnut, who left Egypt for Nubia in a sulk after an argument with her father, back to heaven to be reunited with Re (Sun). When Re retired from the Earth (the end of the sun cycle), he appointed Tehuti and told him of his desire to create a Light-soul in the Duat and in the Land of the Caves, and it was over this region that the sun god appointed Tehuti to rule (moon cycle), ordering him to keep a register of those who were there and to meter out just punishments to them. Tehuti became the representation of Re in the afterlife, seen at the judgment of the dead in the 'Halls of the Double Ma'at'.

The sun cycle and moon cycle are actually equinoxes of the universe. Tehuti was the 'god of the equilibrium' and considered depictions of him as the 'Master of the Balance' to indicate that he was associated with the equinoxes, the time when the day and the night were evenly balanced.

Djehuty is the nominal head of the Ogdoads (group of eight Names of Neter) honoured at the city of Khemenu (Hermopolis of the Greeks), overseeing four pairs of natural synergies: Eternity (Heh/Hehet), Darkness (Khek/Kheket), Water/Potentiality (Nun/Nunet) and Wind/Invisibility (Amun/Amunet).

THE 9 PRINCIPLES OF TEHUTI RELATED TO YOGA

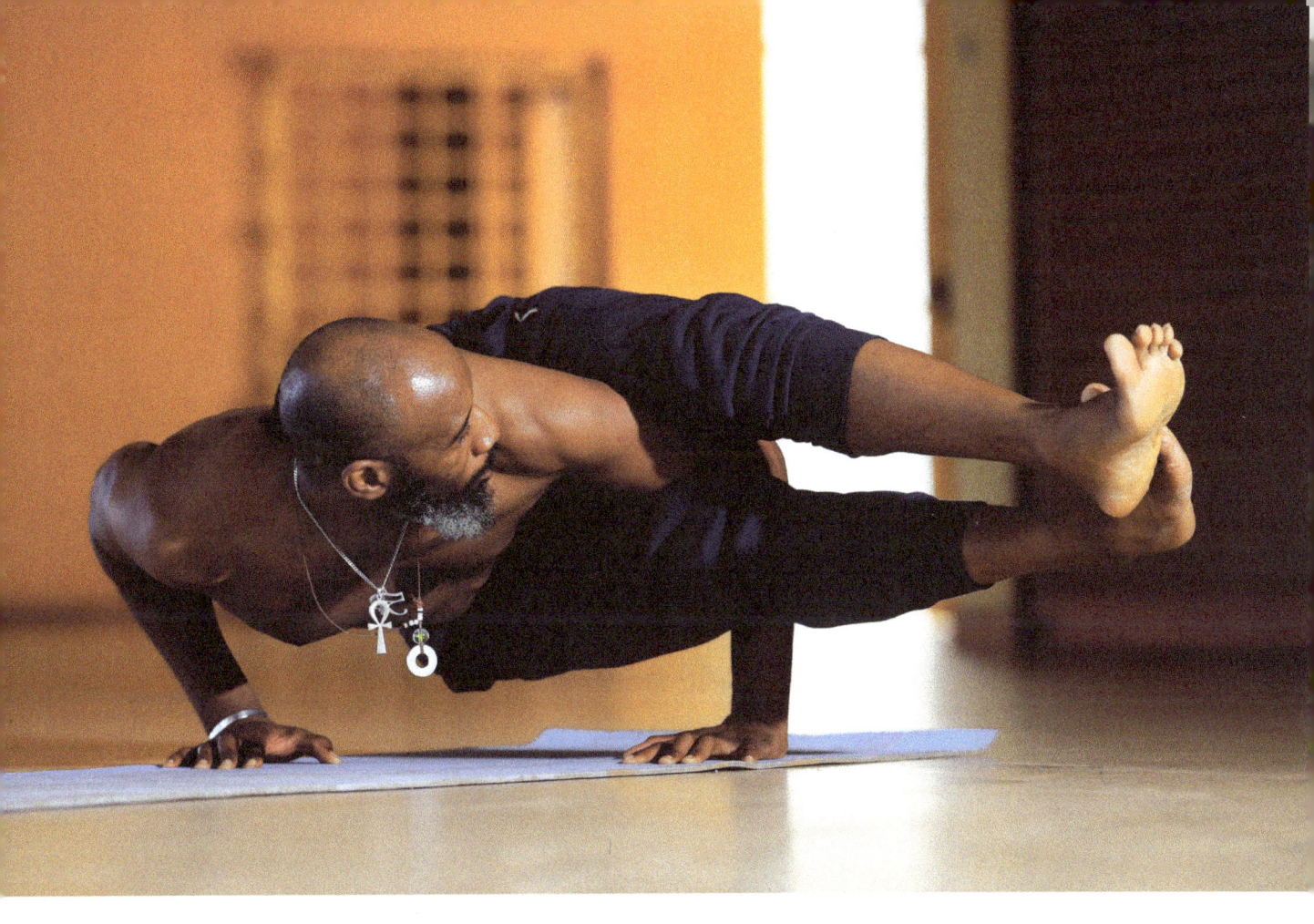

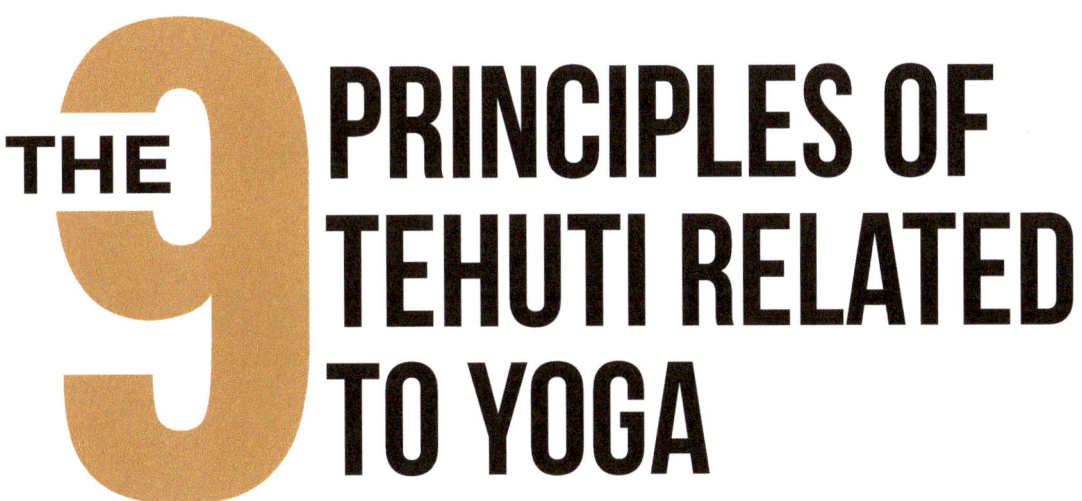

The 9 principles of Tehuti were replaced by what is now known as the Seven Hermetic Laws. Below are the 9 principles, also known as doctrines.

1. Mental (please refer to Meditation exercises, page 125)

We must not confuse mental with mind and mind with general brain function, whose one sole purpose is to interpret impulses, to give and receive information from the various nerves in and on the physical body. Mental or consciousness is beyond the mind. The mind does not merely exist in one's skull but is a pervasive entity of the human being as explained in the 9 principles.

"All is mental and each has a mind" — Tehuti

"Each individual has a mind and is fed by the same mental reservoir, which enables each individual to grasp the laws of the mental and to apply the same to his/her wellbeing and advancement. That's being in touch with a real god.

"With the **ANKH** 'The Master-Key' in his/her possession, the student may unlock the many doors of the mental and psychic temple of Right Knowledge, Right Wisdom and the Right Overstanding, and enter the same freely, using the God mind you have or the mind of mental, which is God. This explains the true nature of energy, power, matter, existence, and why and how all these are subordinate to the mastery of the mind; and that each mind is a slave to mental, the Force of Ether, which controls the action of matter."

Dr Malachi Z York, The Sacred Wisdom

The mental is an area that feeds the mind. The purpose of Afrikan Yoga is to tame the mind and release its potency through the realization and reconnection of the mental reservoir through meditation (stillness) and postures (movement).

Gushing forth clarity with this realization, the practitioner can gain control of their destiny by utilising the principle of mental. Whatever happens to me or does not happen to me is within the mind. One is capable of healing themselves as they now know that sickness and instability arise from the unconscious mind, where there may be a feeling of disconnection with oneself; the 'Self/Being', which is seated in supreme consciousness. Dr Malachi, Amunnubi Ruakh Ptah mention the 'Force of Ether'. This force is inter-layered with our over-soul, which is the Akh (Etheric) you or 'Etheric Body', also known as 'the spiritual plane' overlapping 'the plane of force'. This is channelled through the Mer seat or third eye Arush (Chakra). The plane of material existence is subjected to the plane of force, in the same way, one is able with the use of the mind (re-member: now the mind that is aware of the interconnectivity of all things and knows it is within 'Pa Tempta', 'The All') to magnetize one's wants and wishes; however, be careful what you wish for and use 'Right Wisdom'.

2. Correspondence

"As above, so below; as below, so above" — The Kybalion

This Principle embodies the truth that there is always a Correspondence between the laws and phenomena of the various planes of Being and Life. The old Hermetic axiom ran in these words: "As above, so below; as below, so above."

"In these words, 'as above so below' will mislead you into thinking that there are two directions, when in fact there are no directions at all. Even your own planet is going nowhere, around and back again. So time is going nowhere. And the

grasping of this doctrine gives one the means of solving many blinding paradoxes and hidden secrets of Nature at work in all things."

Dr Malachi Z York, The Sacred Wisdom

There are planes beyond our knowing, but when we apply the Principle of Correspondence to them, we are able to understand much that would otherwise be unknowable to us. This Principle is of universal application and manifestation on the various planes of the material, mental, and spiritual universe — it is a Universal Law. The ancient Smai considered this Principle to be one of the most important mental instruments by which man was able to pry aside the obstacles, which hid the 'Unknown' from view. To ask a question and to be able to see and recognize the answer is due to the realization that all corresponds, is interconnected, and has a relationship. With patience and the application of observation, answers are easier to come by. Afrikan Yoga utilizes the principle in relation to body, mind, and spirit when one is able to form a Sanuy/posture and be aware of the corresponding relationship and effect on the corresponding organ, gland, mental stimuli, and spiritual resonance created by the form in line with breath. The Ancient Smai practitioner led the way and mapped out various movements and sounds, which had their correspondence with internal organs and the planets in our solar system. I give thanks for their wisdom and tireless efforts of self-mastery in order to achieve this and to leave with us a legacy in the movements of Pa Neteru, 'The cosmic principles and forces of nature', Tama-re Smai Taui Afrikan Yoga.

3. Vibration

"Nothing rests; everything moves; everything vibrates" — The Kybalion

This principle embodies the truth that 'everything is in motion'; 'everything vibrates'; 'nothing is at rest' – facts that Modern Science endorses, and which each new scientific discovery tends to verify. And yet this Hermetic Principle was enunciated thousands of years ago by the Masters of Ancient Egypt.

This principle explains that the differences between different manifestations of matter, energy, mind, and even spirit result largely from varying rates of vibration. From THE ALL, which is pure spirit, down to the grossest form of matter, all is in vibration: the higher the vibration, the higher the position in the scale. The vibration of Spirit is at such an infinite rate of intensity and rapidity that it is practically at rest, just as a rapidly moving wheel seems to be motionless. And at the other end of the scale, there are gross forms of matter whose vibrations are so low they seem at rest. Between these poles, there are millions upon millions of varying degrees of vibration. From corpuscle and electron, atom and molecule to worlds and galaxies – everything is in vibratory motion. This is also true on the planes of energy, force (which are but varying degrees of vibration), and mental planes (whose states depend upon vibrations). An understanding of this Principle, with the appropriate formulas, enables Tama-re Smai Taui students to control their own mental vibrations as well as those of others. The Masters also apply this Principle to the conquering of Natural phenomena in various ways. One of the old writers says, *"He who understands the Principle of Vibration has grasped the 'SEKHEM' scepter of power."* With the right vibrational charge, one is able to accomplish anything. To reiterate, this law is the basis for particle physics. It is within this law that resonance is applied to change matter by changing energy. We change things by applying the right frequency or intensity to a subject, object. This is why in Afrikan Yoga we use tones in our movements and also why we Gaanum/Hika Chant as we are summoning light into the body like an invisible laser to heal the corresponding organs. This is also applied to affirmations, as they are commands and decrees consisting of word-sound, tone, visualization, and intensity, all equaling vibrations of will. We are creators of our reality through the vibrations that resonate from our thoughts into the universe.

4. Polarity

The Great Master taught…

"Everything is dual; everything has poles; everything has its pair of opposites; likes and dislikes are the same; opposites are identical in nature but different in degree; extremes meet; all truths are but half-truths; all paradoxes may be reconciled." This doctrine has to be understood in order to bring balance to your being, we are often instructed by master sages to be wary of extremes. Over-stand that extreme ends or poles are one and the same, hot and cold are polarities of degrees of heat. Can you find where hot ends and cold begins? Try this: stand in a room with a fire or a heater and a door exiting outside, and walk from one end of the room to the other just to see where hot and cold begin. This will demonstrate the meaning of duality being the same. It really is down to where you are at mentally. Hard and soft, big and small, positive and negative, like and dislike, and at times love and hate that we experience: all are oscillating vibrations or degrees of mental will, which the Smai student and mystic use to transmute evil into good, a worthless thing into something of use. Remember, mutalub/student: your perception of the world is a reflection of your state of consciousness. The mastery of the principle of polarity or what is known as 'The Art of Polarization' or 'Mental Alchemy' was and is practised by the students of Tehuti. Smai Taui practitioners who devote themselves to this 'Art' will be able to perform a transformation of polarity within themselves at will and therefore change the polarity of others. As was taught by Amunnubi Ruakh Ptah, turn "evil into good". In relation to Smai hanuaat movements or ragulaat exercises, the Smai student avoids extremes so the stretch should always be in the bounds of comfort and devoid of competition with class members or with self (Ego). The stretch with the use of 'Mental Alchemy' will transmute your feelings towards a movement or Sanuy/posture, creating positivity where there once was a negative attitude that created a barrier to achieving the movement.

5. Rhythm (please refer to Hudu/Movement, page 91)

The Great Master taught…

"Everything flows out and in, everything has its tides, all things rise and fall, the pendulum-swing manifests in everything, the measure of the swing to the right is the measure of the swing to the left; rhythm compensates. To swing to and fro you need a point of origin and a fixed spot, as to where the cord hangs from, and the first movement to start the swing. Yet all of this is in The All. This is a physical principle; a motive principle."

This principle of rhythm recognizes the sacred truth of universal law of the passing away and the coming to be of the circular flow of things; "What goes around comes around" (but not always the same way). That "trouble does not last always" and that "joy can be found in the morning". These old African phrases are embodiments of rhythm illustrated by the pendulum swing.

In Tama-re Smai Taui Afrikan Yoga this principle has to be understood by the student/practitioner. The aim is to attain self-mastery and be the holder of the pendulum where you control the rate, speed and eventually suspend swinging to achieve a level of balance between polarities. This at times is unconsciously done, however, when consciously done, that's when the master in you appears.

On a physical level, many Afrikans now living in the West suffer from 'Rhythm Disease'. Many are no longer in tune with their bodies and the subtleties of their soul. So are unable to dance the womb dance or the movements of Pa Netert Tefnut and Het-Heru as can be seen in various Carnivals or 'Bashment', dancehall and African dances today.

I have witnessed the embarrassment first hand when a sister or a brother could not flow rhythmically with the elements around them. Jarred by computer screens, western clothing, 9-5 stress laden city lifestyles, many now copy dances that only mimic movements inspired by joyous living in the sun. The movements become vague and almost unrecognizable to the traditional durational movements of adoration coming from Nomes and villages throughout Afrika.

They are remnants of powerful healing tools of the spirit, mind and body.

Afrikan Yoga removes your stiffness and releases energy flow throughout the body to such an extent that you are able to be aware of your flexibility and your potential to be fully mobile. Reclaim your rhythm and dance more in adoration and gratitude of your life, your ancestors and your divinity.

6. Cause and Effect

"Every Cause has its Effect; every Effect has its Cause; everything happens according to Law; Chance is but a name for Law not recognized; there are many planes of causation, but nothing escapes the Law" — The Kybalion

"Nothing manifests in the effect unless it is in the cause."

Amunnubi Ruakh Ptah

The doctrine of cause and effect is that nothing is left to chance, chance and luck are illusions, and all things are interrelated by a cause that will manifest an effect that becomes another cause. There are various degrees of this law in all dimensions, and nothing escapes the law, as a student you may well be a master if you over-stand this law. For most are subject to cause, but are unaware of it and its effect; so are controlled, manipulated, and pawned in 'the game of life'. However, you may use this law to become movers and even rulers in the game of life where you move and make things happen by will. It is said that nothing escapes this law as you are still subject to obey the law on higher planes of existence. However, you may become masters, rulers, movers, and shakers on your plane of existence. This principle applied to Smai is the understanding of movement and breath. Its cause is the desire, the will and the posture; and it affects the mental, physiological, and spiritual planes. Study each Sanuy/posture within this book to find the effects of them in order to master imbalances in KHAT (body), KA (spirit), BA (soul), KHU (mental) you.

7. Gender (please refer to Taful Sanuy, pages 117 and 123)

The Great Master taught…

"The doctrine of Gender works in the direction of generation, regeneration and creation. Everything and every person contains the two elements or doctrines within him or her. Every male thing has the female element also; every female contains the male doctrine."

It has been said that "spirit has no gender". So when you move beyond physical forms and physical thought processes, gender is non-existent as your polarities are viewed as one. In the womb, genderization is formed in the second trimester and appears where one forms their spiritual and mental interactions (ref Afrikan Holistic Health by Dr Llaila O Afrika). During your creation of physical person(s) in this period as a fetus your sex, mental, and spiritual preferences are also formed; and this is heavily influenced by your parents' interactions, state of mind, nutritional intake, and times of solar and lunar positioning. In the west, there is confusion where gender-swapping is actively encouraged with truly little understanding of 'Gender Principles'. The result is mental and physical violence on the populace by the populace, we unconsciously and consciously hurt each other in this state of ignorance.

Male and female principles are our means of communication, creativity, and harmonizing all aspects of our existence on this plane. All physical beings, objects, and even laws are governed by the principle of gender.

In our cosmology, our explanation of the sciences called mysteries, we communicate via

TA MU NEFU SET [Earth Water Air Fire], which is the Feminine principle. **1. Think 2. Feel (Receive) 3. Process 4. Act.**

TA NEFU MU SET [Earth Air Water Fire] is the Male principle. **1. Think 2. Process 3. Feel (Receive) 4. Act.**

It's important to note that when engaging in movement and stillness, you are having a relationship with these principles within and without your person, and to over-stand them is to know when they are in effect in your being in order to know what being is communicating with you. When communicating with the feminine energy as a male, you will switch to TA MU NEFU SET, which is [Think Feel/Receive Process Act].

When communicating with the male energy, you switch to TA NEFU MU SET [Think Process Feel/Receive Act]. Now, men, take note: a man thinks first, then feels while a woman feels first, then processes. When speaking with a woman, you had better tell her how you feel first. The same concern for the ladies: you better tell a brother what you think prior to how you feel. This will help you avoid many unwanted arguments (however, some arguments are not to be avoided as they assist your understanding and growth as long as you are observing your feelings and self, you can tell what principle you are speaking in, and where the person you are conversing with is coming from). Disharmony can be caused when one is unaware or ignores the facts of this great principle. The mutalub/student is free to express the masculine and feminine principles in the form of 'Shen' and 'Sham', hard and soft. Inverted and extroverted applied in Afrikan Yoga as the Gender principles relate to the Sanuyaat forms, while at the same time they are fused in the one being as there is no gender. This is reiterated in the doctrines of Tehuti.

"Gender is in everything; everything has its masculine and feminine principles; gender manifests on all planes. Again, there is no real gender except what appears in the physical realm and in the spiritual realm. You are neither male nor female, you are god."

The Sacred Wisdom

8. Growth

The doctrine of growth encompasses all principles of creation. The doctrine of growth and creation has been primarily left out of the 7 hermetic laws. Amunnubi Ruakh Ptah teaches that this principle must make Pa mutalub/the student realize, that all things that exist on the physical plane grew. He uses the term 'created', and this creation created itself out of pre-existing matter or energy, also known as dark matter. Even your god concept grew out of darkness; God is not separated from creation but is a part of it.

"And the root reality of creation is that the very word in itself merely means 'to grow'. As habits grow, thoughts grow, knowledge grows, illness grows, bacteria grows, the mind grows but through information channelled from an etheric cord, the mental, the reservoir of outtellect, and the source from which the mind is fed, intellect. These are realities. Substantial realities, material realities. The universe is a phenomenon of life that grew into existence."

As we see ourselves grow materially and mentally, it also has to be recognized that growth in part can be stubbed. However, something is always growing, and it is for the student to be aware of this growth.

Enlightened travelers take care to leave everything beautifully.

Enlightened speakers take care to explore and explain every leaf.

Enlightened science is self-evident; enlightened discussion – self-fulfilling.

Enlightened holism generates free energy.

Enlightened beings have time for everyone and ignore no one.

They pay attention to every last thing, ignoring nothing.

So they are called enlightened.

Just as the enlightened offer examples to the confounded and the confused,

So do the confounded offer opportunities for the enlightened to shine.

To avoid appreciating exemplary beings or to avoid the opportunity of shining would be a mistake, whoever you are.

Realising this subtle interplay is vital to the learning and burgeoning of right relationships; thus vital to evolution.

27 *Tao Teh Ching* by Lao Tzu

9. Breath

The Smai student practices exercises by which he/

she attains control of the body and is enabled to send to any organ or part an increased flow of Sekhem vital force, thereby strengthening and invigorating the part or organ. He/she knows all that his/her Western scientific brother knows about the physiological effect of correct breathing, but he/she also knows that the air contains more than oxygen and hydrogen and nitrogen, and that something more is accomplished than the mere oxygenating of the blood.

"He/She knows something about Sekhem, of which his/her Western counterpart is ignorant, and he/she is fully aware of the nature and manner of handling that great principle of energy, and is fully informed as to its effect upon the human body and mind. He/She knows that by rhythmical breathing one may bring himself/herself into harmonious vibration with nature and aid in the enfoldment of his/her latent powers. He/She knows that by controlled breathing he/she may not only cure disease in himself/herself and others, but also practically do away with fear and worry, and the baser emotions."

Hatha Yoga by Yogi Ramacharaka

The Smai Complete Breath

The Smai Complete Breath is the fundamental breath of the entire Smai Science of Breath, and the student must fully acquaint themselves with it and master it perfectly before they can hope to obtain results from the other forms of breath mentioned and given in this book. They should not be content with half-learning it but should go to work in earnest until it becomes their natural method of breathing. This will require work, time, and patience, but without these things, nothing is ever accomplished. There is no shortcut to the Science of Breath, and the student must be prepared to practise and study in earnest if they expects to receive results. The results obtained by a complete mastery of the Science of Breath are great, and no one who has attained them would willingly go back to the old methods, and he/she will tell his/her friends that he/she considers himself/herself amply repaid for all his/her work. I say these things now, that you may fully understand the necessity and importance of mastering this fundamental method of Yogi Breathing. Start right, and the right results will follow, but neglect your foundations, and your entire building will topple over sooner or later. Perhaps the better way to teach you how to develop the Smai Complete Breath would be to give you simple directions regarding the breath itself and then follow up the same with general remarks concerning it, and then later on give you exercises for developing the chest, muscles, and lungs, which have been allowed to remain in an undeveloped condition by imperfect methods of breathing. Right here we wish to say that this Complete Breath is not a forced or abnormal thing; on the contrary, it is a going back to the first principle – a return to nature. The healthy savage adult and the healthy infant of civilization both breathe in this manner, but civilized man has adopted unnatural methods of living, clothing, etc., and has lost his birthright. We wish to remind the reader that the Complete Breath does not necessarily call for the complete filling of the lungs at every inhalation. One may inhale the average amount of air using the Complete Breathing Method and distribute the air inhaled, be the quantity large or small, to all parts of the lungs. But one should inhale a series of full Complete Breaths several times a day, whenever opportunity offers, in order to keep the system in good order and condition.

The following simple exercise will give you a clear idea of what the Complete Breath is:

(1) Stand or sit erect. Breathing through the nostrils, inhale steadily, first filling the lower part of the lungs, which is accomplished by bringing into play the diaphragm, which descending exerts a gentle pressure on the abdominal organs, pushing forward the front walls of the abdomen. Then fill the middle part of the lungs, pushing out the lower ribs, breastbone, and chest. Then fill the higher portion of the lungs, protruding the upper chest, thus lifting the chest, including the upper six or seven pairs of ribs. In the final movement, the lower part of the abdomen will be slightly drawn in, which gives the lungs a support and also helps to fill the highest part of the lungs. At first, reading it may appear that this breath consists of three distinct movements. This, however, is not the correct idea. The inhalation is continuous, the entire chest cavity from the lowered diaphragm to the highest point of the chest in the region of the collarbone is being expanded with a uniform movement. Avoid a jerky series of inhalations and strive to attain a steady continuous action. Practice will soon overcome the tendency to divide the inhalation into three movements and will result in a uniform continuous breath. You will be able to complete the inhalation in a couple of seconds after a little practice.

(2) Retain the breath a few seconds.

(3) Exhale quite slowly, holding the chest in a firm position and drawing the abdomen in a little and lifting it upward slowly as the air leaves the lungs. When the air is entirely exhaled, relax the chest and abdomen. A little practice will render this part of the exercise easy, and the movement once acquired will be afterwards performed almost automatically. It will be seen that by this method of breathing all parts of the respiratory apparatus are brought into action, and all parts of the lungs, including the most remote air cells, are exercised. The chest cavity is expanded in all directions. You will also notice that the Complete Breath is really a combination of Low, Mid, and High Breaths, succeeding each other rapidly in the order given, in such a manner that one uniform, continuous, complete breath is formed.

You will find it quite of help to you if you practice this breath before a large mirror, placing the hands lightly over the abdomen so that you may feel the movements. At the end of the inhalation, it is well to occasionally slightly elevate the shoulders, thus raising the collarbone and allowing the air to pass freely into the small upper lobe of the right lung, which is sometimes the breeding place of tuberculosis.

At the beginning of the practice, you may have more or less trouble in acquiring the Complete Breath, but a little practice will make perfect, and when you have once acquired it, you will never willingly return to the old methods.

With imperfect or shallow breathing, only a portion of the lung cells is brought into play, and a great portion of the lung capacity is lost, the system is suffering in proportion to the amount of under-oxygenation. The lower animals, in their native state, breathe naturally, and primitive man undoubtedly did the same. The abnormal manner of living adopted by so-called civilized man, which really means western man – the shadow that follows upon civilization – has robbed us of our awareness of breathing and our natural habits of breathing, and human beings have greatly suffered thereby. Our only physical salvation is to 'get back to nature'. To be grounded and connected with Mother-Father Earth.

Grounding is being present in the here and now, connected to the earth and all things. However, sitting in easy pose or Nefertem posture is grounding.

Meditation is the ultimate grounding tool. Begin with 10 mins of silence and stillness a day and build up to one hour.

When breathing what should I do/visualise/be?

Try your Rhythmic breathing to four. If one counts to four for inhalation, one must use the same for exhalation. If you count to four, then your rest or relaxation will be two counts, also your retention two counts, so that you maintain a 2:1 ratio between inhalation and retention, and exhalation and relaxation. You can build this up to 8 counts when you have perfected and are comfortable with four counts.

There are many things one can visualize during Smai breathing, such as self-healing ailments and areas of the body, including the 'over-soul', concentrating on desired outcomes, etc. However, for now during Smai breathing one should keep the mouth closed, and use the imagination (the will and visualization) to control the passage of air entering the body. Visualize the breath entering the nasal passages and floating to the back of the throat and down into your being, and visualize the expulsion of air back up and out through the nasal passages.

What should you be? Well, be relaxed and either lie down, stand, or sit in a comfortable position with your spine straight and your head erect. The standing position is considered to be the ideal position for a number of breathing techniques due to the fact that the distribution of muscular stress is fairly even throughout the entire body, especially if the head is erect, the back is kept straight, the feet are slightly apart, and the arms hang loosely by the sides. However, you can still do this on the bus or at home.

The breathing technique that improves the co-ordination of several systems of the body is both the Smai Complete Union Breathing technique, which incorporates all three clavicles, intercostals, and diaphragm breathing, 'Fug/shallow, Bayna/mid breathing and Tat/low/diaphragm'. This is where the expansion of the diaphragm, ribs, sternum and lungs come into play by steady, slow and continuous inhalation of air through the nose and an equal exhalation occurring to expel the air keeping the mouth closed.

The Rhythmic breathing technique is used where, again, practice is slow and deliberate/conscious or what can be called 'intelligent breathing', where the student controls the time for inhalation, retention, exhalation, and rest/relaxation, repeating the cycle. With rhythmic co-ordination, both the circulatory and respiratory systems benefit significantly as well as other systems of the body.

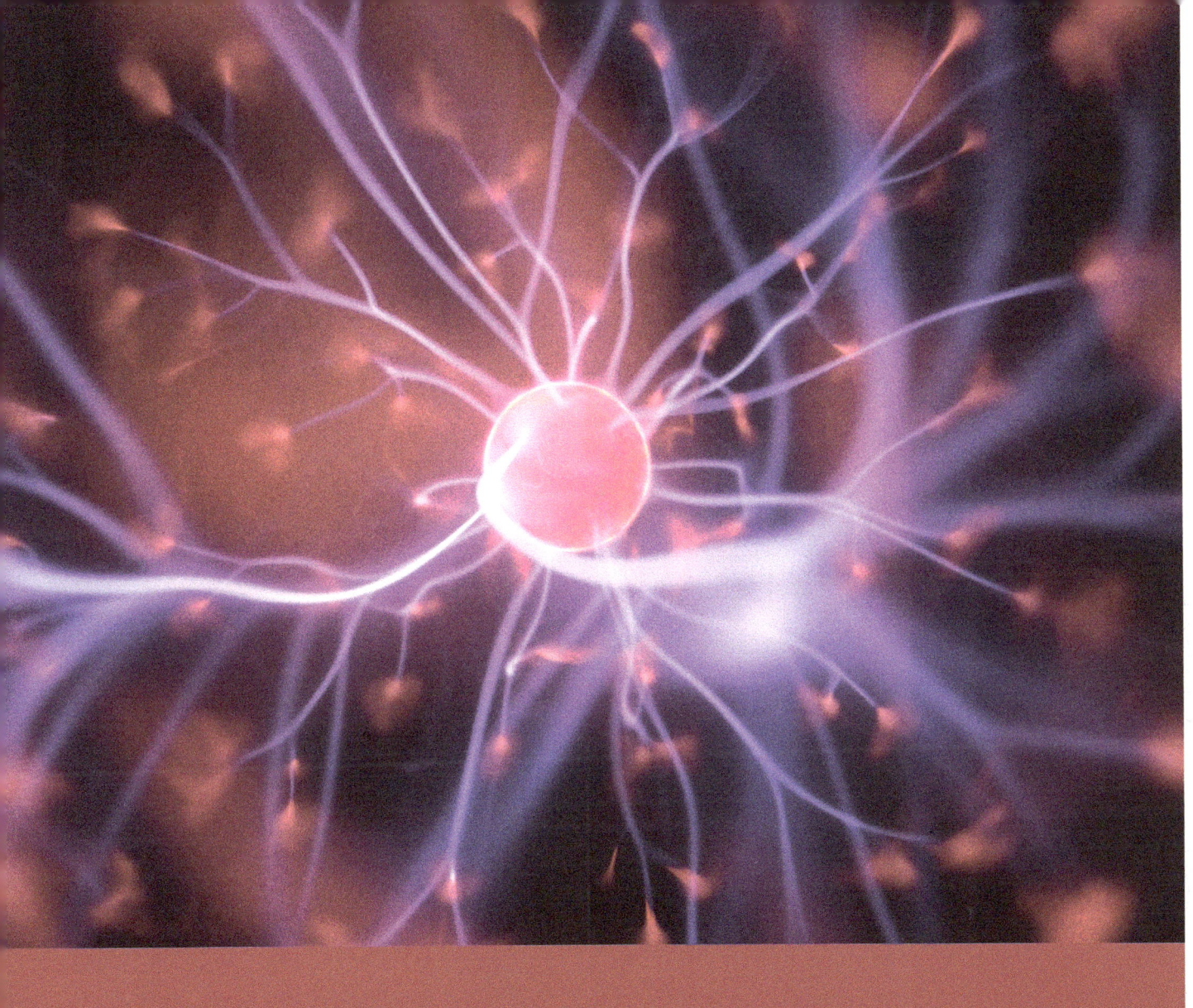

Sekhem...
Spark of Life

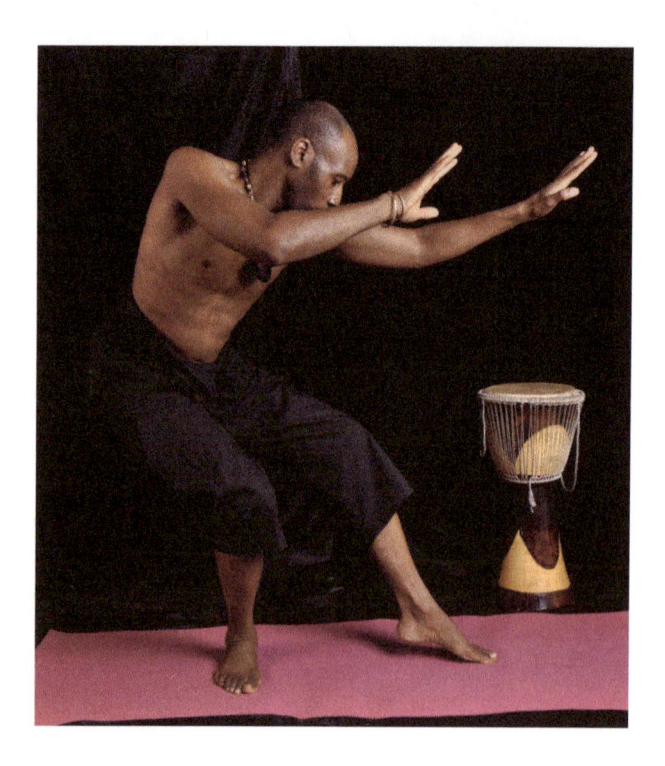

SEKHEM is **SE** — The creative principle, the source of spirit and life force.

SE — The human soul.

KHEM — Black not in terms of colour, tone, or mood but as supreme balance, the true meaning of black. When viewing this meaning in metaphysics and science we have to look at melanin and carbon. Melanin is a conductor and battery, and carbon is the main source of life on this planet.

SEKHEM — 'Absolute energy' commonly named prana or chi, the active principle of life or vital life force.

SEKHEM is the name the ancient ones used for the universal principle, which is the essence of all motion, force or energy, whether manifested in electricity, magnetism, or the revolution of the planets. From the highest to the lowest, moving throughout all of nature in all forms, SEKHEM is the active universal principle also known as the soul of force. It is that form of activity that accompanies all life.

SEKHEM is in all forms of matter, yet it is not matter; it is in the air, yet it is not one of the chemical ingredients of the air. It is in the food we eat, and it is the true nourishing substance of the food. It is in the water we drink, yet not a chemical component of water. It is in the sunlight, yet it is not the heat or the rays of the sun. It is the energy in all these things, the essence and the carrier. Animals and plant life extract Sekhem from the oxygen. Say if we were to breathe in pure oxygen, it would poison us – Sekhem is what gives us life.

SEKHEM is in the atmospheric air, but it is also where air cannot reach. Oxygen and carbon play important roles in the building blocks of life. Sekhem's role is the personification and maintenance of life on a spiritual level, also known as the plane of force.

All physical manifestations have a spiritual counterpart. For example, you. If you were to get sick and had to lie up in bed, your sickness would have manifested in the plane of force/spiritual plane first, then trickle down into your physical being. The plane of force is your 'Black Print', commonly called blueprint. This is the mapping of your being. That's why our Afrikan healers would work holistically, meaning mind, body, and soul, derived from **Ka** spirit, **Ba** soul, and **Khat** body from the principles laid down by the great Master Amun-Hotep student of Tehuti. All things have this black print, so when eating an apple, it is not just the nutrition of the apple you are extracting but the SEKHEM which feeds the spirit as well as the body. This is why organic is so important these days because you cannot create Sekhem in a laboratory like GM food, which is a cloning process.

The air is charged with SEKHEM. The ancient ones knew this, so they would breathe slowly, deeply, and rhythmically. They were able to extract this energy from the air more easily than any other source. The practitioners know that through the practice of the science of breath they are able to store this powerful absolute energy in their nerve centres and use when needed. The miraculous powers of occultists are due to the fact that they are aware of Sekhem and intelligently store this as a clay home would store the heat of the noonday sun or a battery would store electricity, ready to switch on at will. The Smai Afrikan healers were able to generate psychic capabilities using Sekhem, stored in the energy centres, and develop their latent abilities. They exuded the energy of vitality and a healing personality that often radiated strength and would be received as healing when anyone would come in contact with them. They would convey this on anyone they wished, and this is now known as magnetic healing, Reiki healing and Sekhem healing. There are many who have such a personality but are unaware of their source of power.

Sekhem is also a symbol of power; this was a staff of office. The word 'Sekhem' literally means power, Sekhem also symbolizes the stars and is found in paintings with Asar.

Respiration

This the cyclic process of inspiration and expiration. It denotes continuance to do and live again, and again.

Inspiration

As described earlier, taking a breath is known as inhalation or inspiration.

On an esoteric level, inspiration is a divine inhalation of creativity, which Tama-reans, Ancient Afrikans, call out-formation, where you get a download from the outmost-sphere, coming outside of this planet and at times outside of this solar system.

It is also the drawing in of life-force *Sekhem* and the initiating of a life process.

Expiration

Described as the out-breath or exhalation, which is the freedom of illnesses; getting rid in order to renew. It is the motion of completeness, where the cyclic line has been completed to create another circle.

With expiration comes deep relaxation, where one becomes Asar, prepared and ready to resurrect in this world or the next; it does not matter to the Smai/yogi as they are fully aware that the cycle continues.

$4+6=10$ $1+0=1$, which is the oneness of being. Also add a 0 to 1, and you get 9.

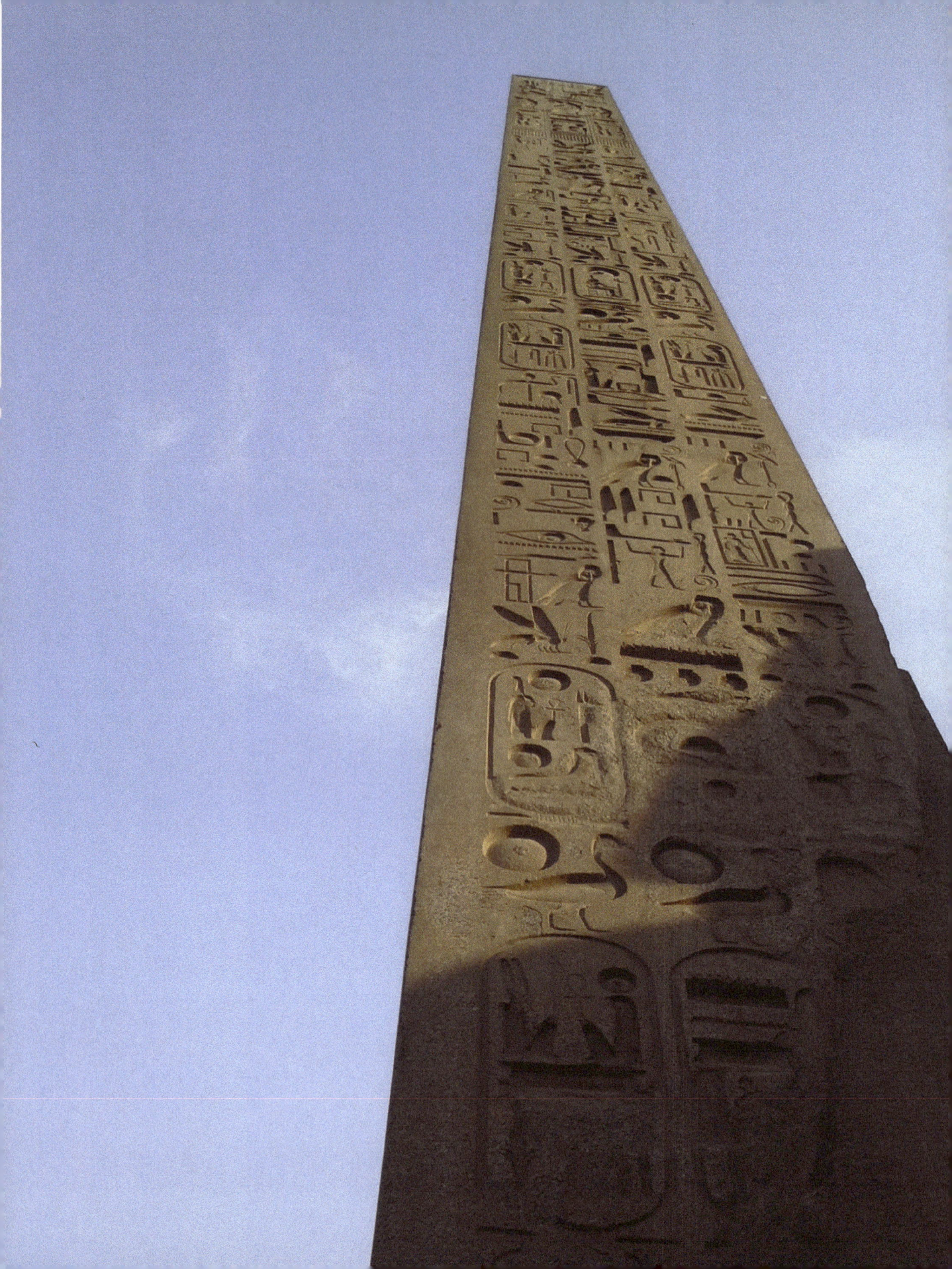

NINE
TO THE 9TH POWER

9 is a sacred number used by the ancient ones; it is also the highest number in the numerical system. All numbers after 9 repeat themselves, for example, zero (0) after nine (9) becomes a one and a zero (10). Number one (1) after nine (9) becomes one and one (11), and two becomes one and two (12), so on and so on until you reach nine, and you go back to zero again. Starting now with a two. Two and zero (20), two and one (21); this continues until you reach nine, and then another zero is added. Afrikan/Nubian moors brought the concept of zero which is a cypher to Europe; this allowed the Europeans to multiply by ten (10) as before that they were counting with sticks and bones called 'Roman Numerals'. The shape of 9 in itself is a 0 and a 1 joined. This is also a computer system 1 and 0 called 'binary'.

The binary number system or binary number code is a system of numbers to base 2 using a combination of the digits 1 and 0. Codes based on binary numbers are used to represent instructions and data in all modern digital computers, the value of binary digits being represented as on/off states of switches and high/low voltage in circuits. The binary system is taken from the Ifa, the divination system of the Yoruba peoples of Ancient Nigeria, who migrated out of the land of Khemet alongside many other families named the Akans during the multiple invasions of the Phoenicians, Greeks, and Romans, and in the last 1000 years, pale-skinned Arabs.

The IFA is an Afrikan spiritual ethic that lays down that one's destiny can only be reached through utilizing three principles:

1. The divinatory processes left to us by the ancestors.

2. Prescriptions of rituals and sacrifices to the spiritual dimensional beings, whose forces impact upon human development and evolution.

3. The moral ethics to which humans must adhere in order to be victorious over oppressive humans and spiritual forces.

(See *The Handbook of Yoruba Religious Concepts*, Baba Ifa Karade)

The binary system has been said to be linked to the Chinese I Ching, which is also a divination tool, however, researches have shown, that the Ifa is at least a thousand years older than the I Ching and actually birthed it.

(See *Ancient Future*, Wayne Chandler)

Looking at these systems, I can also propose that Ifa gave birth to western technological communication through Morse Code and Telegraphy.

Morse Code is an international code for transmitting messages by wire or radio using signals of short and long dashes called 'duration'. The name comes from Samuel Morse who invented the telegraph.

NINE

Composed of all-powerful 3x3 it is the Triple Triad; completion; fulfilment; attainment; beginning and end; the whole; a celestial and angelic number; the earthly paradise. It is an 'incorruptible' number. Nine is also the number of the circumference, hence its division into 90 degrees and into 360 for the entire circumference. It symbolizes the two triangles, which in turn are a symbol of the male and female, fire and water principles.

This symbol is Pythagorean for Nine. However, the ancient symbol is the Egyptian star of creation shown below, where Pythagoras derived his symbol from.

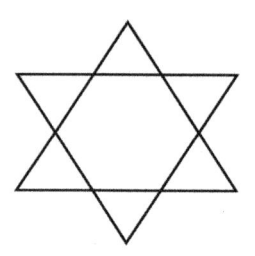

Egyptian star of creation became the 'Magen Dawid'; Shield of David, now known as the 'Star of David'.

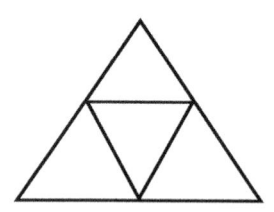

Pythagoras' symbol for 9th to the 9th power.

The average rate of respirations in human beings is 18 (=9) breaths per minute. In an hour, the average, of course, is 18 times 60 minutes, which equals 1,080 (=9) breaths.

In a period of twenty-four hours, one day, the average is 1,080 times 24, which equals 25,920, the time period of the Great Year. (The Great Year was known to all the ancient civilizations of the world and was first used in Tama-re KMT and in India. The ancient ones used this celestial clock to predict events way before they happened. The Tama-reans Ancient Afrikans divided this great clock into 12 portions, creating the zodiac).

As we breathe 18 breaths per minute, the average pulse rate is 72 times a minute; seventy-two is also the time it takes to transit one zodiacal degree in any of the twelve constellations. Seventy-two pulses per minute equal to 4,320 an hour. The number of years in the Kali Yuga, our current epoch, is 432,000.

All the numbers equate to 9 (See Wayne B Chandler's *Ancient Future*).

Dr Malachi Z York raised the awareness of the number 9 and taught extensively about its principles. Here is an example from 'The Holy Tablets':

Holy Tablets Chapter 10

Disagreeableness, Tablet 11 'Nine Ether':

22-39

22. Universal knowledge, called Nuwaubu, informs you, 'New Beings', that there were three creations:

23. Original or primary creation;

24. Evolutionary or secondary creation;

25. And Ghostational or tertiary creation.

26. Primary creation was performed by Nine Ether whose science is Nuwaubu.

27. Nine ether is the combination of all existing gases of nature,

28. Thus, all is in The All.

29. Nothing anywhere can be as powerful as all existing gases.

30. Therefore, nine ether is the most potent power in the universe, 9–9th power of 9.

31. Nine is a very meaningful number. It is symbolic of heaven, hell, and creation.

32. Nine is a number that is symbolic of the three dimensions.

34. Nasswut – abode of mortals,

35. Malakuwt – abode of the Annunagi, Aluhum,

36. Laahuwt – abode of the Most High; and

37. Nine is a number that, when multiplied, reproduces the same figures from up to down and from down to up, and it equals itself.

38. Nine ether was placed in the follicle case of all original Nuwbuns, and it produces the 9 symbol.

39. When the number nine is inverted or perverted, it becomes the number 6…

9 creates 9 of itself; no other number does this. If you do your 9 x tables, you realise the power of nine:

$9 \times 1 = 9$
$9 \times 2 = 18 \quad 1+8 = 9$
$9 \times 3 = 27 \quad 2+7 = 9$
$9 \times 4 = 36 \quad 3+6 = 9$
$9 \times 5 = 45 \quad 4+5 = 9$
$9 \times 6 = 54 \quad 5+4 = 9$
$9 \times 7 = 63 \quad 6+3 = 9$
$9 \times 8 = 72 \quad 7+2 = 9$
$9 \times 9 = 81 \quad 8+1 = 9$
$9 \times 10 = 90 \quad 9+0 = 9$

So it continues. 9 is the infinite number of the universe and the sacred number of all Afrikans ('A free ka' (ns) Tama-Reans, ancient and modern. We are born from 9 Ether, the originator of all existing gases, liquids and compounds.

Nine is the letter I [eye] in the English alphabet, taken from the Greek alphabet, and also links into what is known as the A'IYN principle.

This is a sacred tone translated in Sanskrit as AUM.

The Ennead of
Afrikan Yoga 9 Neteru

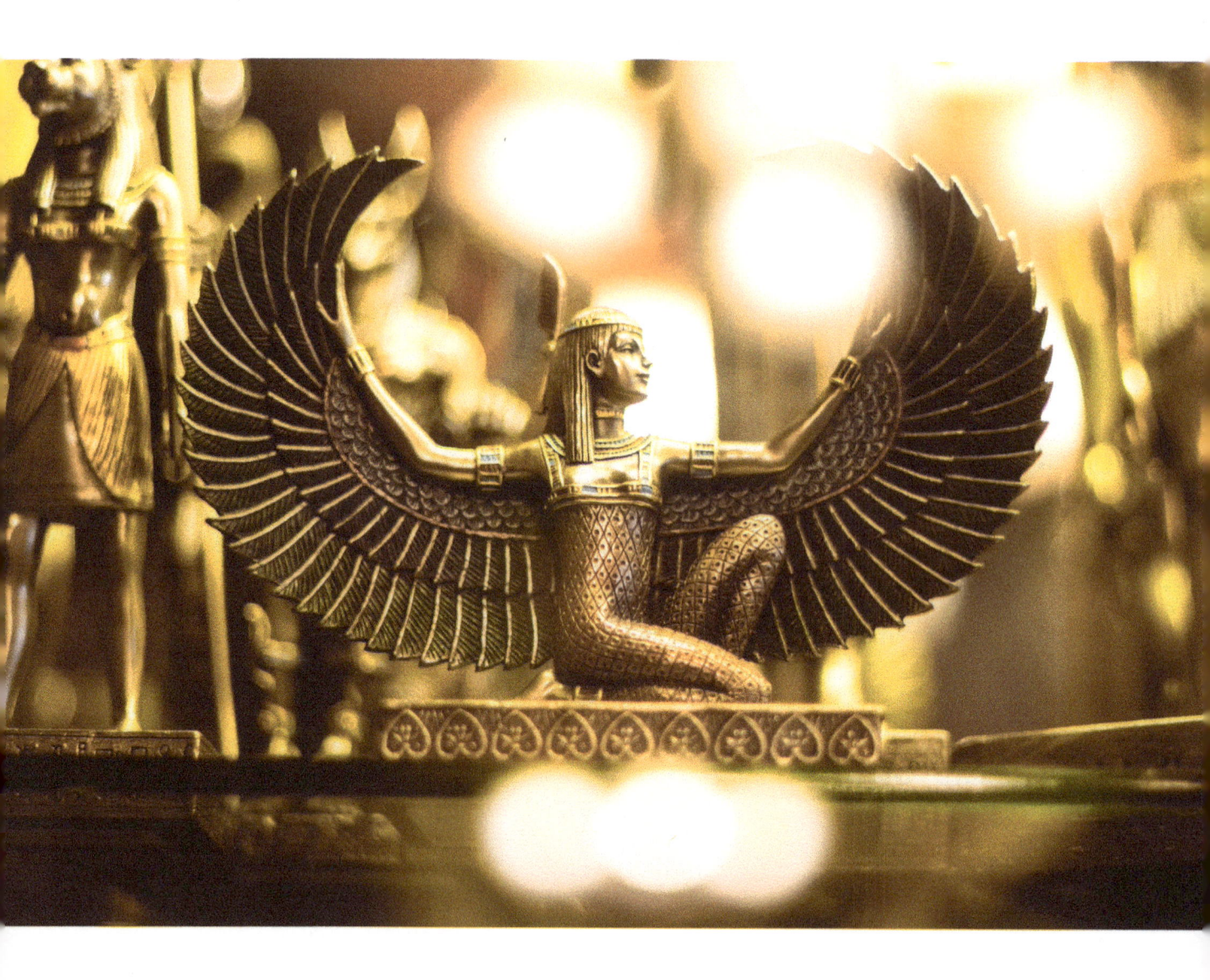

ATUM

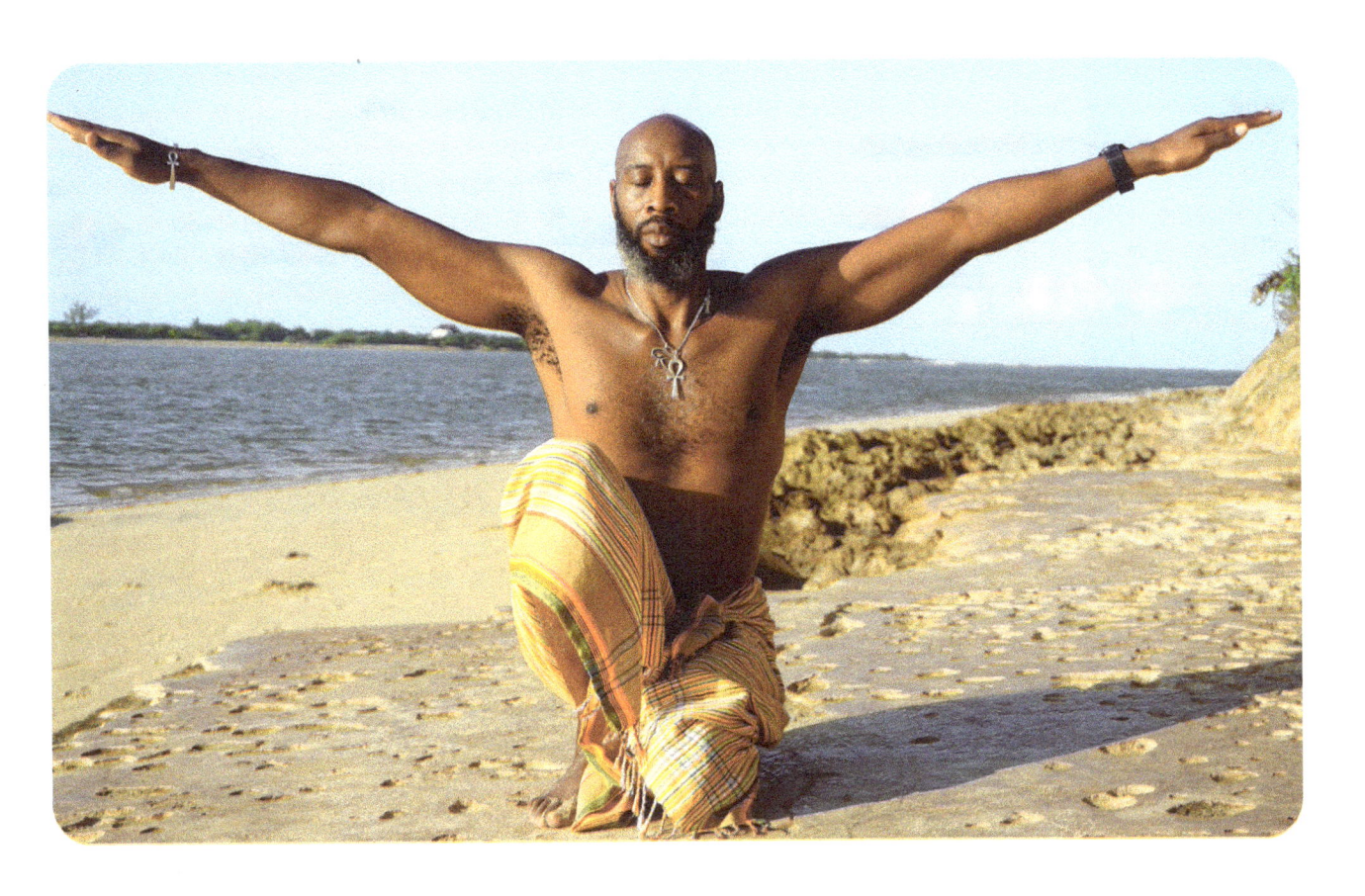

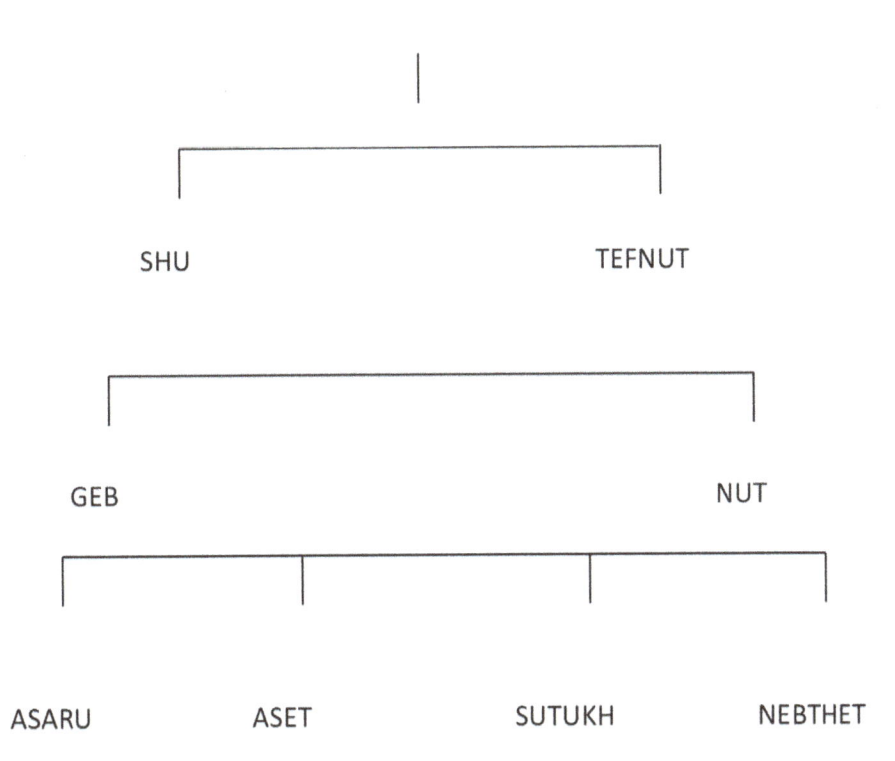

```
            ATUM
              |
       ┌──────┴──────┐
      SHU          TEFNUT
       ┌─────────────┐
      GEB           NUT
   ┌───┴───┐    ┌────┴────┐
 ASARU   ASET  SUTUKH  NEBTHET
```

THE RE-EMERGENCE OF TAMA-RE SMAI TAUI AFRIKAN YOGA | 56

The nine ennead, also known as the company of the deities of ANNU, are the first beings created by Atum/RE.

The word 'Neteru' has been translated as gods/goddesses and deities; this also equivalents to the Orisha of Yoruba, the Eloheem of Judaism, the Annunaqi of the Sumarians, the Allahum of Islam. The Egyptians viewed these beings as ones with great supernatural powers, yet they were finite and mortal. These human deities were endowed with love, hatred, and passions of every sort and many owned more than one title. They represent the forces of nature within all men and women as well as the cosmic forces and principles.

Shu

The Neter Shu, 'The Raiser', according to the cosmology of the people of Anu, was created by a divine sneeze and was the Neter of the sky, and the second member of the Ennead.

He was the firstborn of Ra/Re. He was also known as the Neter of Air and Light, as well as *'The Angel'*. He appears as a human with an Ostrich feather on top of his head and holds a sceptre in his hand. He is the twin brother and consort of Tefnut (secondborn). There are times he appears in the form of a man with his arms upraised.

Tefnut

The Netert Tefnut is known as the third member of the enneads; she is the daughter of Re and the consort of Shu. Tefnut is symbolic of water, in particular, moisture – not only all that is water but also the power of water. Tefnut is the form of a woman, and a woman is symbolic of moistness and an internal creator due to her reproductive seat, her vaginal area as opposed to the male who is dry and an external creator. Water is the symbol of purification and personification as the first form of matter in all cosmologies. Tefnut is a lion Netert, the symbol of courage and intuitive convictions, and was worshipped as a lion; Tefnut and Shu in the form of lions guarded the east and the west horizons. Tefnut in another form personified the power of sunlight.

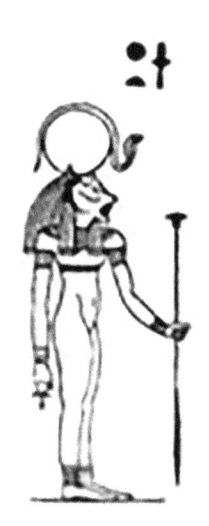

Geb

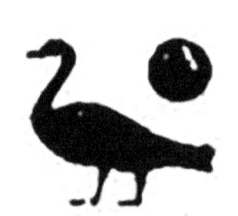

Seb or Geb is the Neter of the earth, and has been known as the 'father of the deities'.

He is sometimes depicted in human form with a goose on his head and because of this symbol, he is also known as 'The Great Cackler', the sound the bird makes when giving birth – this is related to the story of a baby being carried or brought to a family by a goose.

Nut

Nut is the female counterpart of Geb and is the Netert of the sky, and the daughter of Shu and Tefnut. Nut has immersed the many attributes of Female Neters as they have close qualities and characteristics to her.

Set

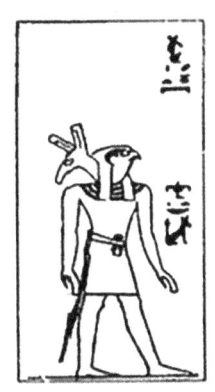

Sutukh or Set was the Neter of storm, night and drought. Sutukh is known as the promoter of illusions, and his name gave birth to Set as in 'setting' sun, which is an illusion, as the sun neither rises nor sets. This leads to further misconceptions around darkness and light, and good or bad which are flags waved fervently by religious doctrines.

This concept of darkness being bad is a very unhealthy ideology for Afrikans, as they are the darkest people on the planet, and this adds to our mental dis-ease.

Many of our scholars still refer to darkness as evil, and this seems to be embedded in our psyche by European education, religion, and ideology. This has to be unplugged, as we can no longer afford to see ourselves as a dichotomy instead of a harmonious whole. When you close your eyes, are you in a state of darkness? Now in that state, there is peace and a true connection with your feelings, yourself and NETERU. This means that the supreme beings and, indeed, the MOST HIGH, reside, in that state. So are you going to tell me, that darkness is bad?

In the Bible, when God created light or said, "Let there be light", which means there was no light until it was said, "Let there be light", in what state was God in?

Yes, God was in the state of Supreme Balance, darkness, triple Blackness (this is all light/true light/not reflected light). Sutukh became Set, the deity of night and darkness, because of his rivalry with his brother (this is the interpretation of the Greeks who stressed the rivalry story, as they are well known for providing us with what is called 'The Greek Tragedies'"– your soap operas of today). We can see similarities in Enki & Enlil of The Gilgamesh Epics, Cain & Abel, Ishmael & Isaac, and Adonijah & Solomon of the Bible, and countless other brother-to-brother battles. This shows that most if not all ideas are based on Egyptian/Afrikan Mysteries. We all have this rivalry going on in our families, so it is a very human story, however, Sutukh was exalted and chosen to ride on the bark of Ra as his defender against Apep, a serpent deity and promoter of ignorance, sleep, anxiety, fear, and doubt. Sutukh, who became Set and Seth in later times, was synonymous with demons, evil, death and crime. Crime because it has been said that Set formed the first police state during the absence of Ausir/Ausar/Osiris, who ruled with benevolence, peace, and justice.

Seth is associated with the language and names of the Hyksos 'Shepherd Kings', the invaders of Khemet, who changed customs and rituals to suit their purpose and were viewed as malevolent. Sutukh, according to the ancient ones, is exonerated and a protector Neter, defender of Ra. We neither see good nor bad; we see what is.

Nephthys

Known as Nebthet, the consort of Set and the sister of Aset, her role as the sister to Aset seems to place a greater value in the cosmology of KMT Ancient Afrika. Nephthys was very close to Asar and Aset. With Aset, Nephthys was the protector of the dead and assisted Aset in finding the location of the 14 pieces of Asar. The goddess was also the mother of Anubis or Anpu, fathered by Asar. A depiction of this story is that Nephthys, in love and adoration of Asar, went to his bed veiled, and Asar, thinking this was Aset, slept with her and consummated Anubu. This is one of the reasons why Set, filled with jealousy, murdered his brother Asar. Nebthet is often shown as a woman with a hieroglyph on her head that formed her name 'Lady of the House'.

Asar

Ausar/Asaru/Usir/Osiris, son of Geb and Nut.

The Neter of crops and vegetation, he is often depicted as green. This is also due to his pure state as a cosmological being who contained less iron content in his body than most Nubians today (Iron when in contact with oxygen and water turns brown, rusts). Asar/Osiris is also known as the 'Lord of the Perfect Black' – this happens to be a title, that Krishna of India carries. The Orion constellation is named after and associated with Ausar/Osiris.

Ausar is known as a solar deity and a pre-dynastic pharaoh of KMT who became the ruler of the dead and the underworld. After his murder, his body was re-membered by Aset/Auset who made the first mummy. He is the equivalent to God, the father, and Jesus of the Christian faith, Isa of Islam, and Tammuz of the Sumerian doctrine (Ancient Babylon doctrine). He is often absorbed into attributes of other Neters, and their attributes appear in his. He is the Neter of death, resurrection, and fertility, as this links to the decay, renewal and rebirth of crops. He taught his subjects, how to grow barley and brew beer, and ruled KMT with peace and justice; to that aim, he travelled far and wide into other lands. He is mostly famed for the story of his death and members of his body being scattered throughout the land, gathered and placed together by his widow Aset, who then aroused him sufficiently to be impregnated and conceive Heru/Horus, who avenged of his father and reclaimed rulership from Sutukh/Set.

Ausar has many forms and another 100 names, too many to mention here; he is often seen as a green man in the form of a mummy wearing a crown and holding a crook, and flail, the emblems of sovereignty and power.

There are certain ceremonies today disguised as Easter, which are ceremonies for Ausar. There is, of course, the opening of the mouth ceremony, performed on the mummy of a pharaoh by the heir, to legitimize the inheritance, and this included purification, anointing and incantations in order to restore the right-mind.

Aset

Aset/Auset/Isis is the female consort to Asaru/Ausar, the daughter of Geb and Nut, and is known throughout Egypt and many cultures as a wise, nurturing lover and mother. The deity Aset is often referred to as 'The Divine Mother' or 'Mother of the Deities', 'The Living One'. She usually takes on the form of a woman with a seat or throne on her head – a hieroglyph of her name.

This Netert is known as Isis (wisdom) amongst the Greeks who also relate her to their deities Demeter, Selene, and Moon Goddess Astarte (star). In Sumeria, she is known as Ishtar and Dina. Aset is Maya in

Buddhism, Fatimah in Islam, and Mary in Christianity. In the Bible, she is mentioned as Ashtoreth, meaning 'star' in 1 Kings 11:5 and 11:33. Aset or Auset or Eset iconography is often that of a mother suckling her child Heru/Horus. This is the original image of the Madonna and child, Jesus and Mary, image of Christianity. Asar, Aset, and Heru are also The Holy Trinity. Aset is known as the deity with many names and appears in all forms of female deities, in particular, Hathor, from whom she has borrowed the cow horns and, indeed, her sacred animal is also the cow; Ma'at, because at times she is also depicted with wings; and also the deity Nut. Aset's fame is of her undying love for Ausar and her courage, and protection of her son Heru that spread far and wide, becoming a story of legend. Aset was worshipped and revered by the Romans and the Greeks, and many temples were built in her name. She was highly skilled in the healing arts and known to pass on her knowledge to the people of the Nile. She ruled with wisdom and justice, while Ausar travelled the world to spread peace. This made Set jealous, as he thought himself a more fitting ruler than Aset.

When Set had cut the body of Asar/Osiris into 14 pieces and thrown them into the Nile, the dedicated Aset searched for each piece with the aid of Nephtys recovering all parts but the phallus, that was swallowed by a fish.

This was after Aset had travelled far and wide to find the body of Asar who was murdered, and his body was locked in a sarcophagus, the trunk of a great tamarisk tree, by Set. She eventually found the Tamarisk tree as a pillar in Lebanon, Byblos, at the Palace of the King and Queen of that country, who had found the enchanting tree floating in the Mediterranean Sea. Auset brought Asar's body back to Khemet, where she used her magic to revive Asar so that she could be impregnated by him, as he did not have an heir via their royal union and an avenger for his murder. This great ancestor Netert was also known as the Mistress of Charms and Enchantment and was able to obtain the secret name of Ra, her grandfather, thus increasing her powerful magic. This was a true power move, as Ra did not give the name away lightly even at the face of certain death. Aset was able to pass this secret name onto her son Heru, as Ra made her promise that he would be the only one she could reveal his secret name to.

Heru

Heru/Hor/Haru/Horus is the famous falcon-headed Neter who avenged his father Ausaru. His depiction as a falcon or falcon-headed man is linked to meanings around his names 'on high', 'the distant one', and 'far away' as well as being a solar deity, who is the Jesus of Christianity and Tammuz in Ancient Babylon, the holy son of God. Heru struggled and fought his uncle Set to avenge his father and to reinstate the rulership placing it back into balance. The story of the wicked uncle or the avenging son is found in many cultures today, even in cartoon movies like 'The Lion King', which is the Heru story. This battle was fought for many days and was a contest of strength, wit and nerve. In the battle, Heru lost an eye, that had to be restored by Tehuti and Het-Heru Hathor, known as the Wadjet. However, this is the contest we undergo in our being as the Heru/ Hero.

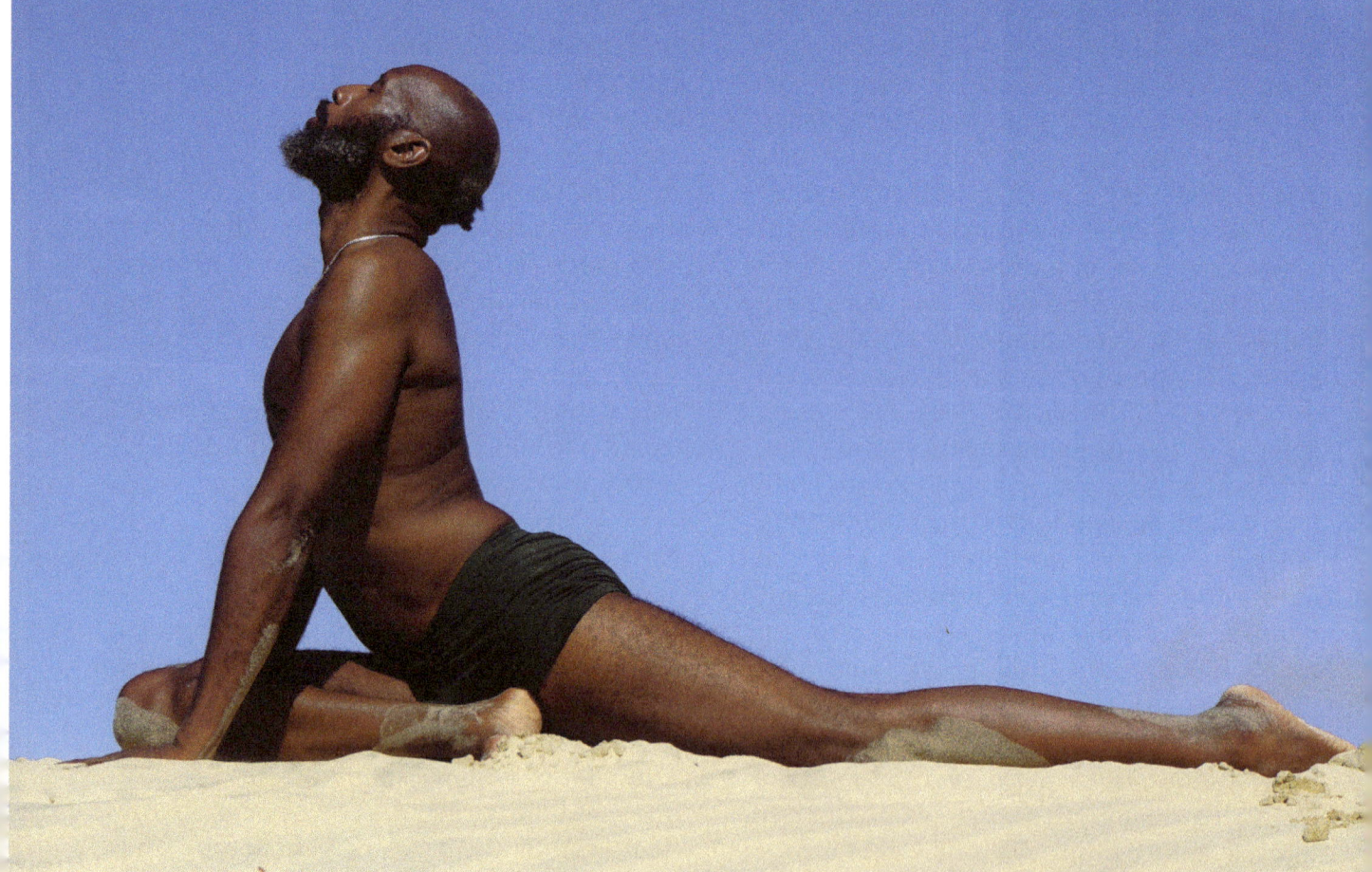

THE 9 Principles of the Human Being

Abdur Kull Tafulataat Wa Baazun Amma Farugun Shil El Kuluwm.

Begin All Prayers and Thinking as a Part of the All.

Ane baruf tased:

I know nine:

El tased kanruhaat:

The nine principles:

Ka, haza izu el nafuslal nee.

    1. Ka, this is the spiritual me.

Khu, haza izu el a'glu nee.

    2. Khu, this is the mental me.

Khat, haza izu el gisum nee.

    3. Khat, this is the body me.

Ba, haza izu el rawuh nee.

    4. Ba, this is the soul me.

Khaybet, haza izu el Khashuhik nee.

    5. Khaybet, this is the plasmatic me.

Akh, haza izu el atherik nee.

6. Akh, this is the etheric me.

Hati, haza izu el maduy galb shil lanee.

7. Hati, this is the physical heart of mine.

Ab, haza izu el nafuslal galb shil laka.

    8. Ab, this is the spiritual heart of yours.

Sekem, haza izu el rameg shil hayuh shil laka.

9. Sekhem, this is the spark of life of yours.

Taken in part from *The Gold Book: The Sacred Tablet of Tama-re,* authored by Amunnubi Ruakh Ptah.

The nine principles of the human being that correspond to the supreme beings, the Enneads, reside in us.

SEKHEM spark of life AMUN RE
AB spiritual heart of mine SHU
HATI physical heart of mine TEFNUT
AKH etheric me GEB
KHAYBET plasmatic me NUT
BA soul me ASARU
KHU mental me ASET
KHAT physical me SUTUKH
KA spirit me NEBTHET

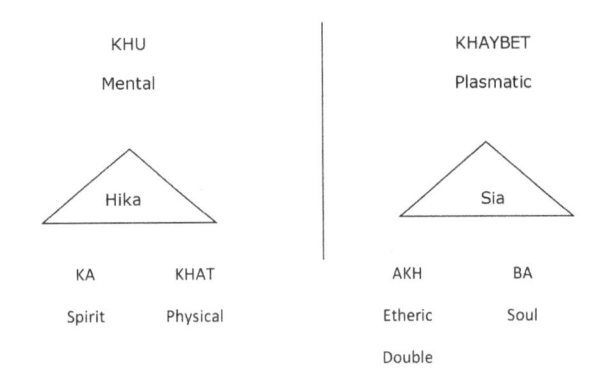

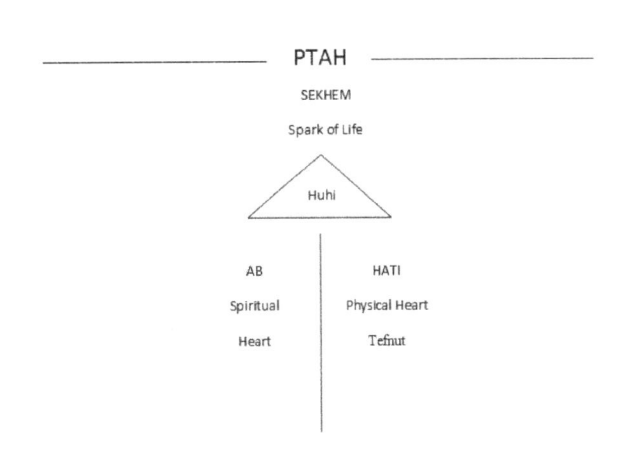

```
      KHU                    KHAYBET
     Mental                  Plasmatic

      /\                       /\
     /  \                     /  \
    / Hika \                 / Sia \
   /_____\               /_____\

  KA      KHAT            AKH        BA
 Spirit  Physical        Etheric    Soul
                         Double
```

```
  ─────────────── PTAH ───────────────

              SEKHEM
           Spark of Life

              /\
             /  \
            / Huhi \
           /_____\

         AB              HATI
      Spiritual       Physical Heart
        Heart            Tefnut
```

The diagram displays the three abodes of Huhi, Hika and the physical realm, Sia.

The 9 principles are interwoven through creation, which is why human beings, unaware, are interconnected with the principle deities throughout time, space and dimensions. They reside within us as us, even though their true power lays dormant within us, awaiting the spark through breath and tone to enliven us once again to bask in the rays of the sun (awareness).

Ptah uses the utterance of tone to create through HUHI. This tone is known as AUM, which became KUWN or KUN as in Kun Faya Kun spoken of in the Koran.

1. In order to create something the Neteru, who are also known as The Ancient Ones, headed by a group of RE called ATUM-RE, ATUN-RE, AMUN-RE, created a state of nothingness, in which to place 99 elements or attributes of this state by HU, Huhi, the eternal, or things on this side of H1.

The Sacred Records of Neter: Aaferti Atum-Re, Amunnubi Ruakh Ptah

Chapter 1. 'The Coming': Scroll 3

*296. In Egypt, **Huhi**, which is **Hu** or **Huwa**, was considered the personification of 'utterance', with which the creator **Ptah 'Ta'**, who was regarded as the creator of the physical world and deity of technology, done its work.*

*297. **Hu** was the utterance or tone, the vibration and pulsation of existence and that which comes to existence within the sacred breath.*

*298. Those things made, that manifest within creation, true growth. **Hu** is that tone from which the creator calls things into being, with **Hika** and **Sia**.*

*299. The original triad of **Ptah, Hika and Sia**. **Huhi** is one of the creative forces of will that constantly accompanies **Re, 'Ra'** the sun deity, the source of life, the sustainer of life, the provider of sustenance in this world, the eternal.*

*300. This highest triad is the triangle with the eye of **Re** in the centre, and the three points of the triangle represent **Atum,** 'the undifferentiated one', in the creation.*

*301. The full disc appearance of the sun in the morning. **Atun** 'the unique one' in life.*

302. The full sun disc at the highest point of the day.

*303. **Amun** 'the hidden one', at death, the sun at its last full disc before setting and making it through the underworld or netherworld.*

*304. These are the sacred names of the three suns, **Shamash, Afsu** and **Utu** of Sumeria, and **Hu, Huhi, Huwa** is the etheric counterpart of the Nether world.*

305. These beings once dwelled in this realm, and now they are guiding forces and controlling forces from beyond this world, working as the involuntary to the voluntary in the human body.

The Sacred Records of Neter: Aaferti Atum-Re, Amunnubi Ruakh Ptah

Chapter 1. 'The Coming': Scroll 1. 296-305

Maulena Karenga, who selected and retranslated the sacred wisdom of Ancient Egypt, coined the work THE HUSIA, which has the two principles, HU and SIA, placed together:

"The title of this text, The Husia, is taken from two Ancient Egyptian words which signify the two divine powers by which Ra [Ptah] created the world, i.e., Hu, authoritative utterance and Sia, exceptional insight. Thus, I have put the two together to express the concept of 'authoritative utterance of exceptional insight'. Given the importance of authoritative utterance and exceptional insight to the moral and spiritual realm and their divine character in Ancient Egyptian theology, Husia appears as both compelling and proper as a title for a text of Ancient Egyptian sacred writings."

From the introduction of THE HUSIA by Maulena Karenga

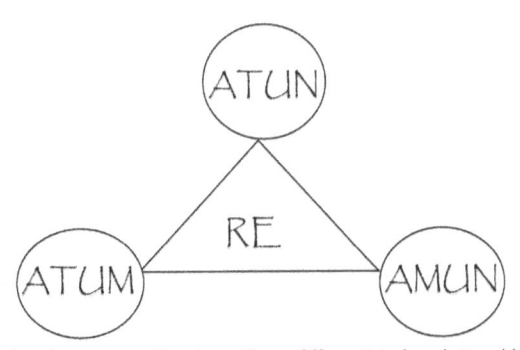

The Three States of Re, Atum 'the undifferentiated one', Atun 'the unique one' and Amun 'the hidden one'

306. Hika is an anthropomorphic personification of miracles, magic, and the manipulation of elements, and chemicals of nature.

307. Hika is one of the two constant companions of Re. The other being Sia.

308. Sia is the personification of perception, shape, form, pattern who work together in Huhi with Hika and make the world of created things possible.

309. So, **Huhi, Hika** and **Sia** are a triad principle of godship, the Neteraat [Neteru], responsible for the consistent and perpetual pattern of that which manifests, in that which is created and made, and that tone or utterance is **Aum,** which later was rendered as **Kun** as in existence or **be.**

The Sacred Records of Neter: Aaferti Atum-Re, Amunnubi Ruakh Ptah

Chapter 1. 'The Coming': Scroll 1. 306-309

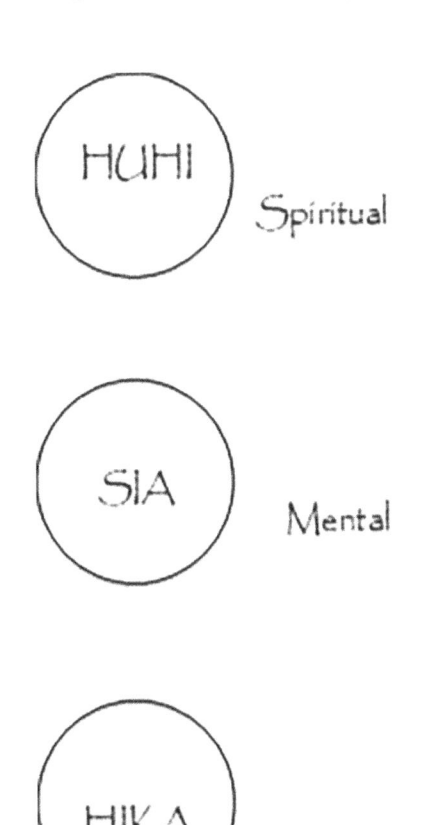

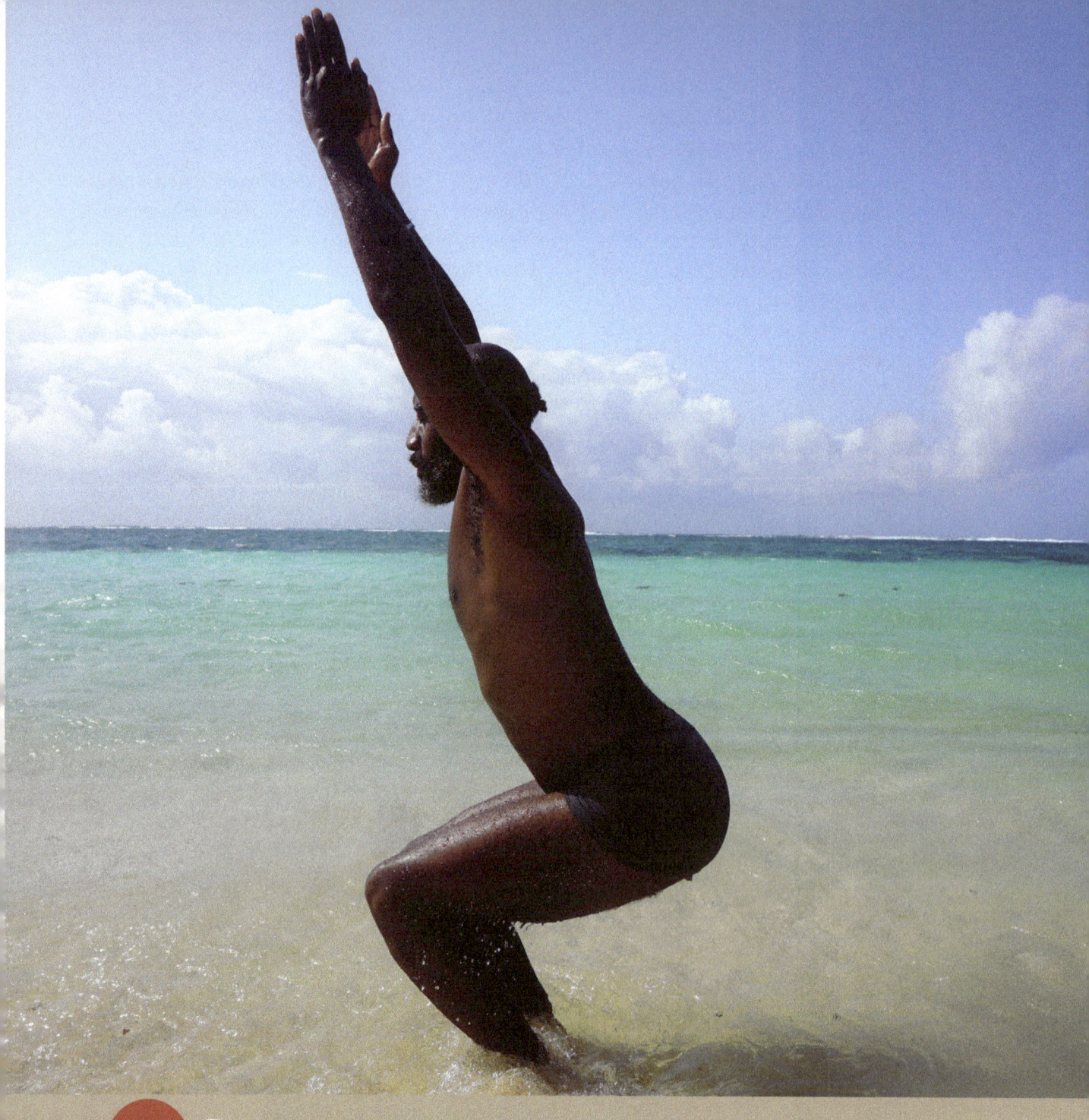

THE 9 PURPOSES OF SMAI/AFRIKAN YOGA

1. Emancipation/Freedom

Freedom gives us the ability to really choose and not feel pressured into doing things that go against our spirit. You have freedom of expression and freedom of thought. Thinking for yourself, you are completely guided by your inner divine self and not manipulated by others. Some are bound by relationships, some are bound by their guru or teacher. Freedom is when one merges into supreme consciousness and is 'one with The All'.

The practice and cultivation of Afrikan Yoga does not only acknowledge freedom but also allows access to freedom now in your life, wherever you are in your life. It enables you to feel the wisdom of Ma'at flowing through your entire being, becoming 'A Free Ka' (Ka meaning spirit).

Many of us will now have to learn to be free; we may find it difficult, painful and unattainable. You can be free by being true to yourself.

2. Action

"Do or Do Not, There is No Try" – Yoda, Star Wars

Earlier I mentioned Ma'at and her divine principles. One of the key principles of Ma'at is that of action. Even though we may have gained intellectual knowledge and understand the maxims, able to repeat chapter and verse verbatim, which in today's society may seem to be acceptable criteria for establishing a group or being accepted by a clique, the experience is the master teacher, which is one of the points of Nuwaubu, the science of all nine ether solar beings (Tama-reans Ancient Afrikans).

It has to be understood, that there is knowledge without thoughts and words, knowledge so abstract that it cannot be taught – only experienced, lived and breathed. The student and the teacher become one in the realization of witnessing this knowledge that is much more than the intuitive self.

Within application, keen observation, perseverance, patience, and compassion for oneself this knowledge begins to reveal itself. The essence of this knowledge is waiting for you and is constantly placing opportunities in our paths to grasp its spirit, and to acknowledge it, to express it, to know it and to be this 'it' as living knowledge. The opportunity arrives in the forms of near-death experiences, trauma or witnessing trauma, or even overwhelming joy.

The ari-action in Afrikan Yoga is fundamental, it just goes without saying as I have been taught. *"Lift up the self by itself for the self is the self's only friend and the self is the self's only foe."* Within this teaching, you find yourself ultimately responsible for self and a recipe for self-mastery through action. Ari, the word for Action, is a principle of Ma'at in line with karma. In Afrikan Yoga, the principle of **Ari** is simply applied as a series of one or more exercises ragulaat (ragul) or postures (Sanuyaat) in combination with Smai breath, gaanum (chanting), istanizaah (visualization) and transformation, in a specific sequence designed to produce specific effects. The ari-aat used in Afrikan Yoga (Tama-re Smai Taui) is thousands of years old. The effects of Ari are greater than the sum of its parts, which is to say these Sanuyaat, as simple as they look, are not to be underestimated for their power to heal physically, mentally and spiritually.

3. Knowledge

"If Knowledge is the key, then ignorance is the door" – Khonsu Sekhem Ptah

"The purpose of acquiring knowledge is to nourish one's character. But one who merely pursues knowledge as an end in itself misses the point of education."

Cai Gen Tan/The Vegetable Discourses by Hong Yingmin of the Ming Dynasty

"Know thyself" is the axiom of the ancient ones written on the pylons of Ancient Egypt. This is an important part of Smai, as knowing oneself is self-empowering.

Many people have accepted "book learning" as the total sum of knowledge or method of knowing. This is unfortunate, as knowing self is true knowledge because it is the means by which you perceive yourself as the microcosm of the boundless universe. Through meditation, you learn this self-awareness, this perception, and you begin to project from within out as opposed to gathering of facts; you develop insight. Through meditation you realize that you can turn yourself inside out, creating your reality. The universe provides for you as you are the universe. Another axiom is: *"As within so without."*

4. Power

Those with true power have no need to flex their muscles as true power is a magnetic force that commands respect by its sheer grace, serenity and influence. It is a manifestation of Sekhem that resonates in all aspects of your life. As I mentioned earlier, many believe the idea of power is a big muscle-bound male or acts of violence. Power exists in your self-image and therefore is a force of spirit. For the martial minded amongst you, hear the words of Carlos Castaneda, *"…warriors are in the world to train themselves to be unbiased witnesses, so as to understand the mystery of ourselves and relish the exultation of finding what we really are."* What Carlos is actually speaking about is freedom, and with freedom, there is power as the two are synonymous. The suggestion is that a true warrior is liberated or free. It is this freedom that gives the warrior power. Warriors must purposely seek change.

The Smai practitioner is a spiritual warrior, and the ultimate realization of the spiritual warrior is to flow into wholeness. This flow is with humility and transcendence, that which is personal.

Personal power or acts of empowerment

Afrikan Yoga/Tama-re Smai assists the process of reclaiming your power by involving you in self-reliance through these steps:

1. Acceptance of self and who you really are, overstanding of your issues and manipulations.

2. Awareness and acceptance of your life, and what you have created.

3. Acknowledge and appreciate your gifts, talents and abilities from the core and separate this from the satellite superficiality that clogs your progress.

4. Be responsible for your life and no longer sit in a pain body being a victim and blaming others.

5. Pro-actively self-heal and seek further changes in your life. The very reason YOU do this work on yourself is because your life transfers into another level of personal power, living free from victim patterns and actualizing your free will.

5. Love

Ashug/Love is represented by Hathor/Het Heru.

Ashug is a synergy, a glow that we feel; it's a light that reflects off us. It's not something that we can use, it's something that uses us. WE do not make love, create love, nor can we do these things; the best lovers are the vessels of love. The love that we feel is actually the connection to all things from all things. Ashug is the interwoven thread from the supreme conscious right down to the unconscious, but when we are in a state of unconsciousness, this love appears as something that we own, deserve and barter with, and if things do not go our way, this perception of love turns to hate. Actual ISHQ/ASHUG awakens you to your spiritual higher senses, where one sees with an inner seeing, hears with an inner hearing and feels with the inner heart/spiritual heart. The lover accepts what is, and with acceptance, there is no resistance, no pain, and no conditioning. "The All is I am." This is a person, who carries light and rays of sunshine about their being; they heal by just being present. Ashug is fundamental to the practitioner of Smai – without this purpose, he/she is an empty vessel. When we open ourselves up to love, we receive abundantly what the universe has to offer us. The universe is father/mother to us all. When we open up to the universe and universal love, we begin to receive the guidance and assistance to pass through the 'bottlenecks' and 'needle eyes' of life with ecstasy and ease.

6. Transcendence

"A person is said to be established in self-realization and is called a Yogi (or mystic) when he is fully satisfied by virtue of acquired knowledge and realization. Such a person is situated in transcendence[3] and is self-controlled. He sees everything – whether it be pebbles, stones or gold – as the same."

(Bhagavad-gita 6.8)

Afrikan Yoga/Smai is a tool for developing transcendence, moving from one state to the next mentally as spoken about in the Hah Kah, the Hermetical laws of polarity, vibration, etc. You gain transcendence through expression, not repression.

That is to say, the road to transcendence is not a self-righteous priesthood road where one pushes down their feelings, lusts, angers, jealousies, etc., but by expressing these feelings and going into them deeply and purely. Once these feelings are experienced and explored, they can be left behind, transcended. Transcendence is the complete awareness of illusion and not feeding into the illusion created by the ego. In a state of detached observation, you rise above or move from so-called problems, challenges and hurdles; reassigned to a state of higher consciousness, free from

---

3 Transcendence is also the ability to see things as they really are.
Please refer to the 10 Virtues of Ma'at **'Learn to distinguish the real from the unreal'** (page 25).

constraints and reactionary behaviour that often habituates your life's moments and events. Transcendence is not being a person full of airs and graces with an attitude of "I am above you", or placing yourself as a judge of others, but recognizing the divine in all people. *"A person is said to be still further advanced when he regards all – the honest well-wisher, friends and enemies, the envious, the pious, the sinner and those who are indifferent and impartial – with an equal mind."* (Bhagavad-Gita 6.9) You see all as one and these labels cease to exist. Why? Because you know through your own experience. You are rooted and grounded in self-acceptance, self-love and your spirituality, and therefore are free to allow yourself to be. When truly accepting, you allow others to be also, no longer feeling the need to control their lives, but allowing yourself and others to experience life as it unfolds. In the form of transcendence, you become a Heru who is able to control his lower nature (ignorance, hate, jealousy, etc.) and become one with his higher self, 'Asar', one who is able to resurrect from a dead state of ignorance to a state of eternal life on the djed pillar of wisdom. This brings a state of hetep/peace.

7. Wisdom

"Wisdom is often found in the chambers of meditation" – Khonsu Sekhem Ptah

The Smai adherent looks to Tehuti (the male principle of wisdom) and Ma'at (the female principle of wisdom) in meditation and within their internal structure, and within their bones and bone marrow, where the DNAs of our ancestors are kept.

This is the intuitive knowing, when one says, "I feel it in my bones." In combination with this knowledge, the 'Ari' action(s) of the aspirant is the personification of wisdom. Wisdom is not merely the manifestation of inspirational words and truths. It is also the divine, inspirational actions of truth that promote harmony.

We are in a time of much devastation and ill will, the age of ignorance and destruction, however, the spell of sleep is lifting. The sleeping giant within us is awakening and the principles, such as wisdom, are now being activated to bring forth the supreme balance of Black Light that covers the full spectrum of waves, colours, moods, dimensions and realms. For all sits in Blackness, even this planet is surrounded by Blackness. You know this once you venture out of this atmosphere, you know this once you close your eyes in meditation and feel the comforting nurturing womb of the universe expanding into nothingness, into Pa Tempta, The All. This is the realization of the wise, that *'nothing is all things'*, a complete cypher to which you are a part, interconnected and one with ALL. Through meditation, you may say, "I am not this body, I am not this thought or action." There is no identification with "things", and this is where you become nothing, interconnected to all things and vessel for the manifestation of the divine. It's a paradox. Have you ever asked someone what they are thinking after a break in a conversation and they say, "Nothing"? One or two things may be happening. One, they have drifted into subconsciousness. Two, they are unaware of the many thoughts that possess them. They are unable to slow down the process through feeling and then to communicate it clearly, concisely and honestly, devoid of judgment, with love – the type of love we equate with when a parent instructs a child. This wisdom is intricately linked to feminine values and, once tapped, used in all relationships. So when they express their thoughts, it is authentic and self-aware.

8. Joy

Joy is a feeling of relief, of abundance, of achievement, of love, of heat that rises up your spine and fills the well of consciousness, that expresses itself in a smile, in laughter, in tears, and also in silence. Joy must be in all actions that you do, whether it is work, play or relaxation. When you do things joyfully, you find that the task is effortless. Where there is no joy or enjoyment, you will soon find a reason to stop. A person can perform work or do their job joyfully with very little pay, as long as they find joy in the tasks, they will stick to it. A person can receive high amounts of payment for a job and not enjoy the job. They will soon give that job up or endure it painfully. Joy is a motivating force that will manifest abundance. Be joyful in all things.

9. Truth

"The Truth shall make you free" once you have dropped the dead weight of lies, then you are able to soar to heights beyond your expectations. Truth does the miraculous work of laser cutting and healing. There is also recognising truth as a resonance of healing – why should one feel pain when they hear or see, or feel the truth – the pain comes about through resistance of what is. In a Sanuy/posture, your body does not lie, it knows its limits in the now and it places you directly with now. (You may visualise yourself doing amazing things with your body; in your moment of now, the truth is, the body will do a fraction of the things that you visualise. This is ok, keep visualising as your present truth will eventually change in due time.) The Smai/Afrikan Yoga student learns to recognise truth through practical experience and not just as an intellectual experience of movement and form. This in turn applies to your recognition of truth in your daily life where you feel as well as observe and analyse. The continued practice then becomes more feeling, and the fluidity of truth now begins to flood your being. There is now a synapse jump from the analytical "I want, I need, but I can't have" to spirit, feeling and knowing, "I have, and I am abundant". With this awareness, there is hope for future expansions on any dimension you wish. For truth in no way should weigh heavily on your heart. Truth sets you free.

Afrikan Seats of Light...
THE 9 ARUSHAAT CHA KA RA(S)

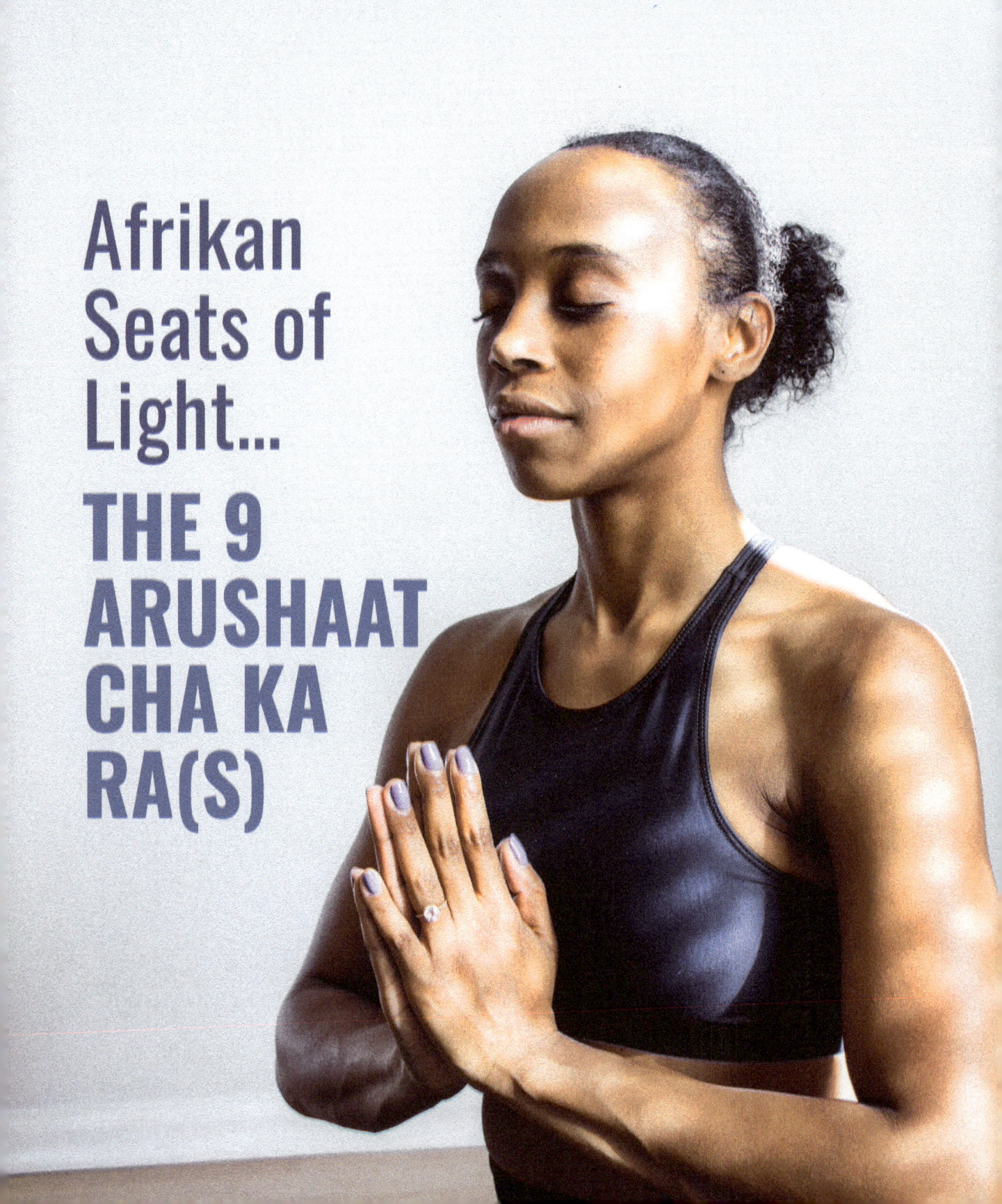

The Arushaat (seats) in the body are focal points of exchange, where the psychic, spiritual and physical planes of existence entwine to produce an exchange of energy. They work as transformers changing the subtle sekhem into physical energy that flows through the meridian lines in and out of these seats, connected to our personal atmosphere or energy field, known as your Aura. Auras are called 'Tepi Hesp' by the Ancient Afrikans. The arushaat act as vortexes, whirlpools of great energy; and they are nine in total in the Afrikan and not seven as we are taught by the Indian Hindu yogis. The melanated Afrikan can perceive cosmic gamma waves right down to radio, TV and electric waves, in fact, the whole light spectrum, where Caucasians perceive the light spectrum of the rainbow, which is seven bands, also known as the visible light spectrum or standard photon band. Therefore, the highest attainment of Caucasian body type is seven chakras but many may only attain 6. The reason is that the seven bands or visible light spectrum placed in a prism will break down into six colours. This is in line with the body type. The perception of the visible light spectrum and the electromagnetic spectrum is interlinked with the arushaat and melanin.

Arushaat's Connection to Melanin

Melanin from mela means 'black'. Afrikans are not taught about melanin in school. This would empower them to think for themselves, and, indeed, to perceive their dark skins as an asset rather than a liability. It would open their minds to their own divinity and seeing themselves as living sun entities, very aware of life and their connection to the universe. The subject of melanin is key to the understanding of Afrikan spirituality, chakra activity and capabilities that appear to be superhuman and even supernatural. Dr Carol Barnes, Dr Llaila O Afrika, Jewel Pookrum and Richard King speak intensively on Melanin; and their works, studied with fervour, will serve you well in the understanding of Melanin and, indeed, the understanding of the A Free Ka (n) people.

Carol Barnes tells us in his introduction to the book **Melanin: The Chemical Key to Black Greatness:**

"The Black Human is blessed by nature in that he or she is endowed with a highly functional chemical that regulates essentially all bodily functions and activities. The Black Human is distinguished from other human species in that he or she tends to have a higher number of organs and body systems that contain high concentrations of a chemical that is BLACK in colour. This Chemical is called MELANIN and is responsible for manufacturing and sustaining life.

"MELANIN is located in important areas of the BLACK HUMAN such as:

– Central Nervous System

– Autonomic (Automatic) Nervous System

– Peripheral (outlying, surface) Nervous System

– Diffuse Neuroendocrine (Glands) System

– Visceras (Major Internal Organs)

Because of its pervasive presence in the organs, nervous systems and glands cited above, you would expect MELANIN to serve some vital function or nature would not have incorporated it into these systems!!!"

What Carol Barnes is saying in this last statement is that MELANIN is the key to the bodily systems of all people on the planet. As it is more prominent in Afrikans, western scientists are not raving about it and have suppressed this information about melanin serving a vital function. This is hideously amazing hence the exclamation marks.

There is much more to be said about melanin, however, I want to direct you to the Arushaat/(C)ha-ka ra(s) and their connection to melanin; why Afrikans have nine and why I have mentioned that Afrikans perceive higher states of consciousness naturally. Melanin is a key component in the ability to do and actualize this.

Blackness is all light, all energy and, indeed, absorbs all light. You only have to read and listen to scientists as they explain Black Holes. The study of photography and chromatics can also explain this as the subject of photography teaches you about light spectrum and colours, which are forms of energy that are perceived.

Carol Barnes explains this eloquently: "MELANIN is BLACK simply because its chemical structure will not allow any type of energy to escape once that energy has come into contact with its structure." Carol Barnes goes on to say, "The Human eye sees the colour of an object as light reflects from the surface of that object. If no light or energy is reflected, then that object will appear to the eyes to be BLACK in colour. If all of the energy is reflected from the surface of an object, that object will appear white in colour.

"If an object appears red in colour, then that object is absorbing all energy around it except the red energy, which is reflected away from the object.

"Light energy from the sun or artificial sources like your indoor light bulb or vibrational sounds from your stereo, all causes melanin to be black in colour, for instance, a light wave leaves the sun or your stereo in the form of energy particles and/or vibrational sounds and travels in space until it contacts the melanin structure in your skin, and other areas of the body, where it is absorbed by MELANIN."

Melanin: The Chemical Key to Black Greatness

This is to say that we perceive energy not only through the human eyes. According to scientists, who now attest to what the ancients have taught, we are made up of fine particles of energy that are constantly vibrating; and this is the make-up of our bodies, our skin (skin colour and tone), limbs, organs and glands.

Corroborating this with Carol Barnes' research, it is sufficient to say Afrikans are absorbing and perceiving (not reflecting) high amounts of light, colours, sound, and wavelengths of energy, making them darker in pigmentation but also giving them access to higher states of energy through the photon or visible light spectrum. The visible light spectrum perceived by Afrikans covers electric power, radio, TV, microwaves and infrared. Other frequencies of light perceived by Afrikans are ultra-violet, x-rays, gamma rays and cosmic rays. This is interlinked with glandular activity alongside the Arushaat (the seats of light that are within the body).

Note: Afrikans of dark pigmentation must beware that this is a manifestation of outer melanin that makes up the colour and there are a thousand other forms of melanin within the body, with chemical, physical and personality properties. This is not an opportunity to tell yourself that you are superior to anyone else. Lighter skin Afrikans also possess the uniqueness melanin gives. Europeans may be deficient in melanin, yet some use the little they have to greater effect than Afrikans. There is also the problem of Afrikans becoming sick because of the melanin becoming toxic due to inadequate diet, lack of exposure to sunlight, detrimental music and thoughts. The quality of melanin is related to lifestyle and spiritual practice.

"The black dot is an ancient symbol for blackness, it is the black seed of humanity, archetype of humanity, the hidden doorway to the collective, unconsciousness-darkness, the shadow, primaeval ocean, chaos, the womb, doorway of life."

Dr Richard King, *African Origin of Biological Psychiatry*

"The circle is the symbol of the crown Chakra. The circle sometimes contains a single black dot to indicate the first principle, the source of existence. The circle represents spirit and the whole cosmos, everything that is. The dot is the seed of a new life, the limitless given form."
Cassandra Eason, *Chakra Power for Healing and Harmony*

The sekhem, the ancient name for energy that flows through the meridian channels, is assisted by melanin that allows the energy to flow fluidly, easily absorbing and conducting energy. The Afrikan Smai practitioner uses this knowledge to fully engage in what is happening. Utilising this in their psycho-physical states the Afrikan yogis transform themselves at will and converse with the Ancient Afrikan scientists, the Neteru, who emerged out of blackness and were the first to study and clearly understand the principles of the universe. They did this by studying their own blackened state, a methodology they leave with us today for we are told to 'know ourselves'. We can do this by studying the outer and inner blackened state through meditation.

The nine arushaat overlap and feed into each other. They also represent the various dimensions of existence. Within the chart, one can find the glands of the endocrine system that affect growth and nerve action.

THE 9 ARUSHAAT/CHA KA RA(S) TABLE:

Arush	Location	Organs/glands	Symbolism, dimensions, existence	Colours	Musical notes
9. Ikh Ether	Head	Pineal	Mental/ Meditating	White/ Black	All 8 keys together
8. Mer Spirit	Brow	Hypothalamus	Intellect/ Thinking	Violet	C
7. Shiru Breath	Nasal	Pituitary	Air/Life Breathing	Indigo	B
6. Sehem Mucous	Throat	Thyroid/ Parathyroid	Protecting/ Verbal Communication	Turquoise	A
5. Heper Blood	Heart	Thymus	Healing/Curing	Green	G
4. A'b Solar Plexus	Diaphragm	Adrenals	Heating/ Circulation	Yellow	F
3. Tekhet Liquids	Navel	Islets of Langerhans/ Pancreas	Life/Nourishing	Blue	E
2. Tchet Sacral Semen, Ovum	Groin	Ovaries/Testes	Carnal/ Reproducing	Orange	D
1. Setekht Base Soul –E-motion	In between perineum & base of the spine	Prostate/Uterus	Lusting	Red	C

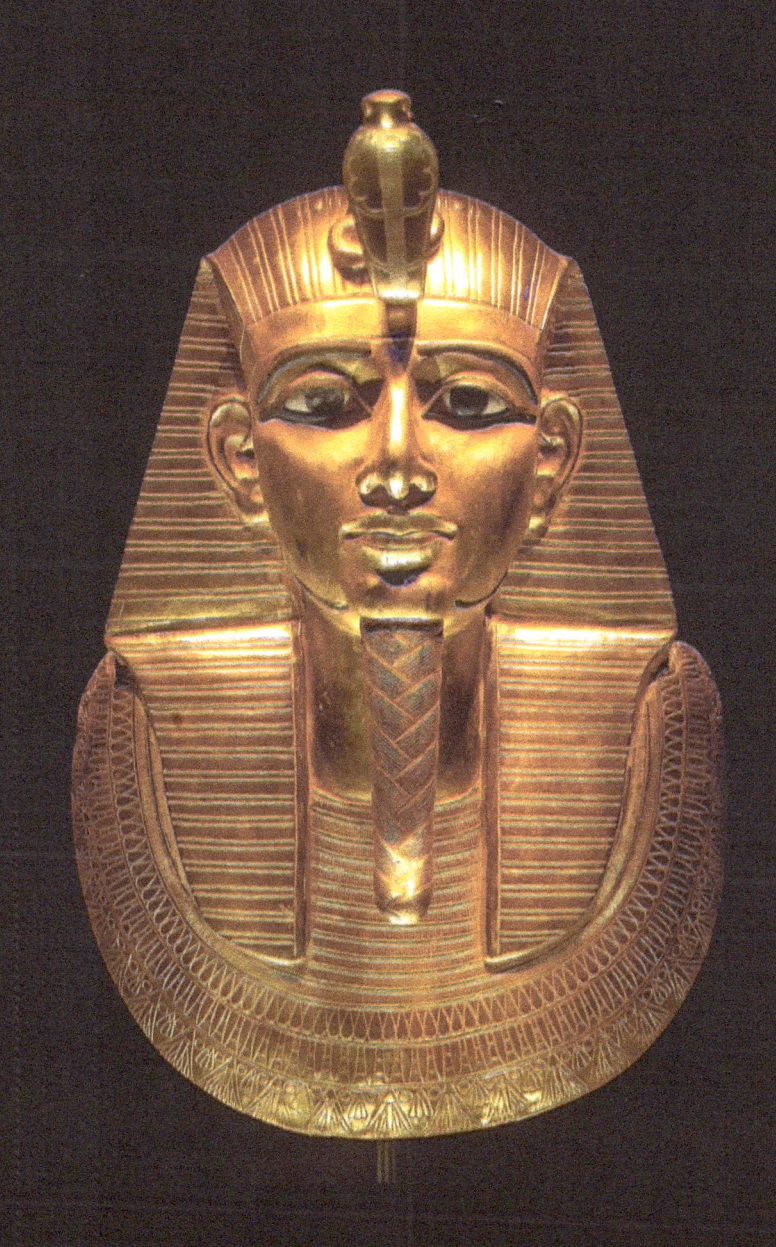

PERSONALITIES OF UNBALANCED AND BALANCED ARUSHAAT/ ENERGY CENTERS

SETEKHT Prostate/Uterus

UNBALANCED

Insecure
Fearful
Feels unstable
Feelings of lack/Poverty consciousness
Financial issues
Inability to let go and trust
Possessive
Disconnected from the environment
Feeling of isolation
Feels drained
Ungrounded
Wants to leave the body
Escapism

BALANCED

Secure
Feelings of abundance
Prosperous state of mind
Feels safe
Ability to trust
Connected to the earth
At one with the body
Grounded

TCHET Semen/Ovum

UNBALANCED

Obsessive behavior, including sexually
Inclined to jealousy and revenge
Dissected/separateness
Unable to satisfy creative expression
Unable to accept self
Craves what he/she feels cannot have
Inner child is in pain

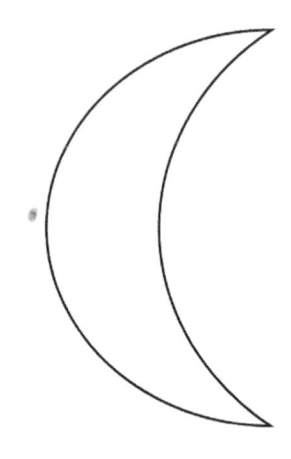

BALANCED

Sexuality is integrated into his/her life
Opportunities of creative expression are in every part of his/her life
Connection with others
Loves self
Secure in self
Spontaneous/flowing with life
Healed inner child

TEKHET Naval

UNBALANCED

Anger
False pride
The need for recognition
Selfish motivation

BALANCED

Dissolved anger
Feeling of connection
No longer needs to manipulate others
Self-importance fades
Positive ego identity
Selfless service develops

AB Solar Plexus

UNBALANCED

Not centred
Open to disease
Lacks vitality
Inability to commit and maintain actions and intentions
Unable to break habits
Addictive
Possessive
Seeks personal power
No consideration for the common good
Lacks integrity and honesty
Revengeful and angry
"Me first"
Feeling of being a victim
A blamer

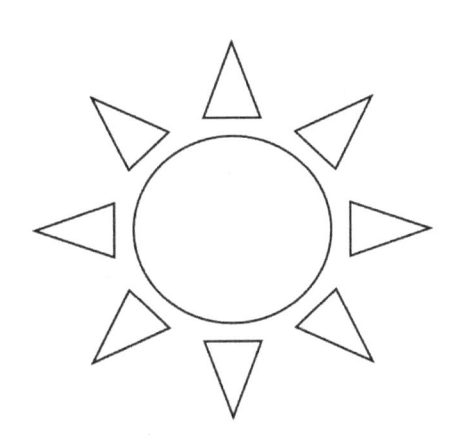

BALANCED

Centred
Vitality and health
Personal power
Wisdom and strength
Ability to commit, persevere and maintain
Flexibility/Ability to change
Reflects on inner sounds
Unattached
Ability to consider the common good
Integrity
Love and compassion radiating from within

HEPER Heart

UNBALANCED

Emotionally attached
Dependent relationships
Neediness
Selfish
Self-hate
Jealousy and envy
Weak immune system
Feels alienated from life
Lack of purpose

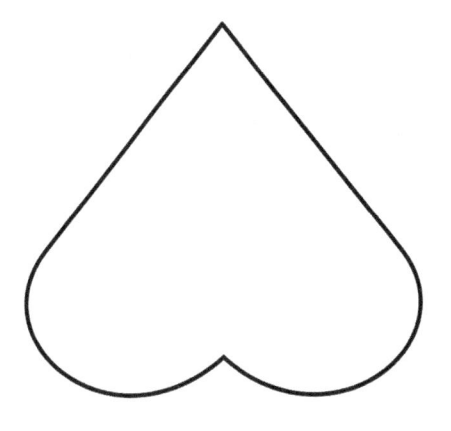

Sacred Spiritual Heart that points to the divine

THE RE-EMERGENCE OF TAMA-RE SMAI TAUI AFRIKAN YOGA | 78

BALANCED

Male and female energies synchronized
Balanced relationships
Compassionate detachment
Self-love
Strong immune system
Ability to heal oneself and others
Committed to the universal plan
Contented
At peace

SEHEM Throat/Thyroid

UNBALANCED

Fear of communicating
Inability to express self
Delayed reactions
Hesitant in interactions

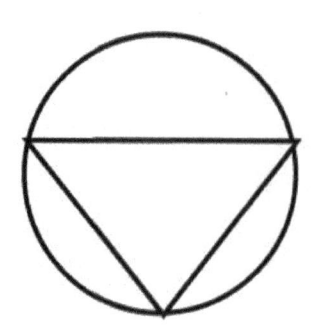

BALANCED

Ability to fearlessly communicate and speak one's own truth
Quick intelligent response
Self-confident in interactions

SHIRU Nasal pituitary

UNBALANCED
Blocked creativity
Inability to sense danger
Sees no way out
Struggles with thoughts
Disoriented
Memory impaired

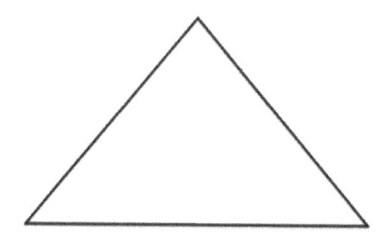

BALANCED

Clear thinking
Even clarity
Control of breathing and heart rate
Senses energies
Open, alert and intuitive
Accesses memory and all dimensions of time

MER Brow/Hypothalamus

UNBALANCED

Has to analyze everything
Needs physical proof
"I believe it when I see it"/ overly cynical
Fixed in mind and intellect
Non-accepting
Caught in emotional pain

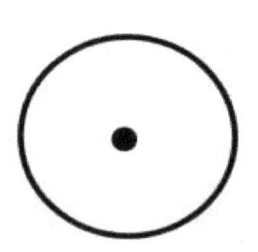

BALANCED

Intuitive knowing
Sensing abilities
Mind serves higher self
Inner hearing, inner seeing and inner feeling
Can listen inside and get an answer

IKH Crown/Pineal

UNBALANCED

Only aware of physical reality
Unable to move beyond the five senses
Distrusts and negates (ancestral) higher forces
Has to take control
"Do it alone" mentality
Alienated from soul
Negates inner being

BALANCED

Experiences realities beyond the physical receptors of the five senses
Open to all realities of existence
Ability to perceive, feel and experience soul
Ability to connect to inner being
Trusts higher powers

- Only the well-centred, well-grounded and well-balanced can dance, revolve, and spin along beautifully
- Real understanding lightens the heart
- Calm unshackles frenzy grip
- Throughout the unfolding of each day, enlightened ones never lose touch with their inner centre and transcendence
- Only when well-rooted in the certainty of spiritual intuition can one realize freedom and transcendence
- You might as well ask, how can a person with responsibility act without a sense of calm and understanding?
- Inattention indicates instability
- Agitation indicates a loss of centre

26 Tao Te Ching by Lao Tzu

To my mental and physical efforts, I add the potential of my spiritual self.

Its qualities permeate affairs. Its powers flow through my entire being.

By Amunnubi Raakhptah

The Twelve Principles of an Initiate

1	Kindness
2	Concentration
3	Meditation
4	Praying
5	Fasting
6	Exercise
7	Self Healing
8	Cheerfulness
9	Patience
10	Silence
11	Unselfishness
12	Humbleness

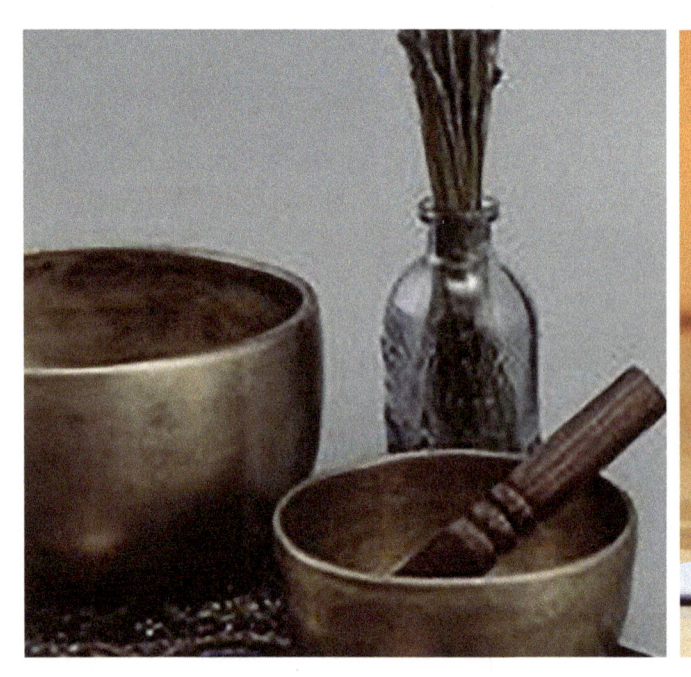

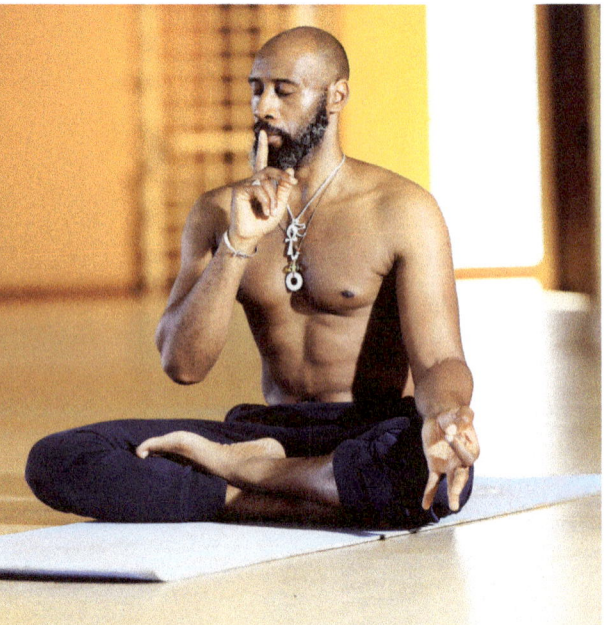

HIKAU
WORD-SOUND AND POWER
The Science of Sound Healing

Holy Tablets Chapter 1: Tablet 7: 72-73

72. After a universe collapses in its centre or contracts, it expands, which is an explosion called a 'Big Bang', producing the sound KHA, from which the word 'KHALUG', 'create', comes…

73. It is the same sound that each being that comes into this world makes as the womb contracts to yield for birth. The baby gurgles out, 'GHA' and 'KHA', remembering the sounds of chaos in creation. As one thing comes into existence, it fractures other things to form itself.

TONES

When you make a tone, you summon forth light from the spinning wheels/Arushaat, that are set in motions due to resonating sound to come and fill the corresponding organs with life, movement and revitalization.

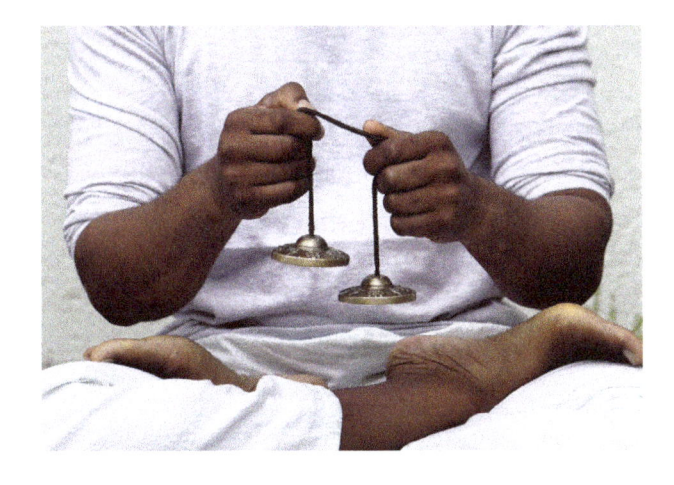

Afrikan Yoga movement and forms, what we call Hanu and Sanuyaat, are enhanced with the use of tones. The tones are used with the breath, coming from the diaphragm up into the back of the throat and, exhaled or expelled out, to create the sound. In the Om or the Ankh, the sound comes from the diaphragm up into the back of the throat and is exhaled with the mouth slowly closing. Now the tongue is touching the roof of the mouth, allowing the sound to vibrate into the nasal area. This links into the Shiru Arush opening the Mir Arush (third eye).

The nine tones that correspond to the nine parts of the human.

A (pronounced AAAAAH) Healing and stimulating tone for the lymphatic system and digestion.

AH (pronounced AAAAAAUUUUUHHH) Healing and stimulating tone for the respiratory system.

HAH (pronounced HAAAAAAAAHH) Healing and stimulating tone for the heart, gall bladder and liver.

KAH (pronounced KAAAAAAAAHHH) Healing and stimulating tone for the pineal, kidney and bladder.

E (pronounced EEEEEEEEEEEHHHHH) Healing and stimulating tone for the pineal, the pituitary and nasal *(arushaat)*.

O (pronounced OOOOOOOOOHHHHH) Healing and stimulating tone for the pancreas and spleen.

U (pronounced UUUUUHHH) U is a healing, stimulating tone for the stomach and large intestine.

OM/Aum (pronounced AAAAAAUUUMMMMM) Allow this tone to vibrate into the nasal cavities. OM is a healing and stimulating tone for the entire nervous system and all *(arushaat)* energy centres. Resonating from the solar plexus through to the nasal seat.

Ankh (pronounced AAAAAAUUUUUNNNNNNNKHH) Allow this tone to vibrate into the nasal cavities. Ankh is a *healing, stimulating tone for the heart and life resonance on all planes.*

Hikau (Mantra) for Psychic Self-Defence and Transformation

Psychic Self-Defence

Heru Wadjet Udjat (repeat as many times as you wish), "Calling on the all-seeing eye of Horus."

For a psychic attack of any kind; also for the promotion of strength and vigour.

Uplifting the consciousness

Sa-Su-Temu – Heru-Hakenu (repeat as many times as you wish).

"Making an offering to the son, to Temu-Horus, the praised one."

To lift the consciousness into realms of mental and super mental activity that ranges far beyond the physical.

Immediate protection

Erta Na Hekau Apen Aset (repeat as many times as you wish).

"May I be given the words of power of Isis." Can be used to initiate immediate aid and protection; it can also be used to provoke intuitive hints for action for anyone facing any form of threat, be it from physical danger or disease, or of a psychic or spiritual nature.

Strength of Will and Purpose

Asaru – Djedu (repeat as many times as you wish).

Incorporating the Djed principle. Used to promote the strength of will, wisdom and over-standing, also to nurture spiritual transformation and growth.

Happiness and Good fortune

Nefer Neter Wedineh (repeat as many times as you wish)

"The perfect God grants life."

Repeating this attracts protection, inspiration, happiness, good fortune, and bonding with higher forces. It can also be used with a Neter's name drawing on the attributes of the chosen Neter.

The transformation from a Human to a Super Human Mantra

Ankh (repeat as many times as you wish) Tone: AH UN KH A (pronounced AAAAAAAUUUUUUUNNNNKHHAAAA)

Three Names of Ptah

Ankh Ptah Sekhet (repeat as many times as you wish)

Asaru (repeat as many times as you wish)

---

[1] Om/ Aum is also short for Amun (pronounced AAAAAAAUUUUMMMMUUUUNNNNNNN)

For a protective force on all levels of human activity and a process of transformation from a human to a superhuman.

Tone: **A SAH RU (U)** (pronounced AAAASAAAAAAHHRUUUUUU)

Pa Faatuh/The Opening

Hikau used to open the spiritual channels and raise the spirit in the abodes of the three suns ATUM, ATUN and AMUN. This hikau can be useful prior to, during and after meditation. This hikau can also be used before your practice.

Aum Atum Aum Atun Aum Amun Aum Kuluwm Aum

Amun

To Awaken the KA/spirit

Tone **AUM MUN** (pronounced AAAAAAAUUUUMMMMUUUUNNNNNNN)

Sound Colors

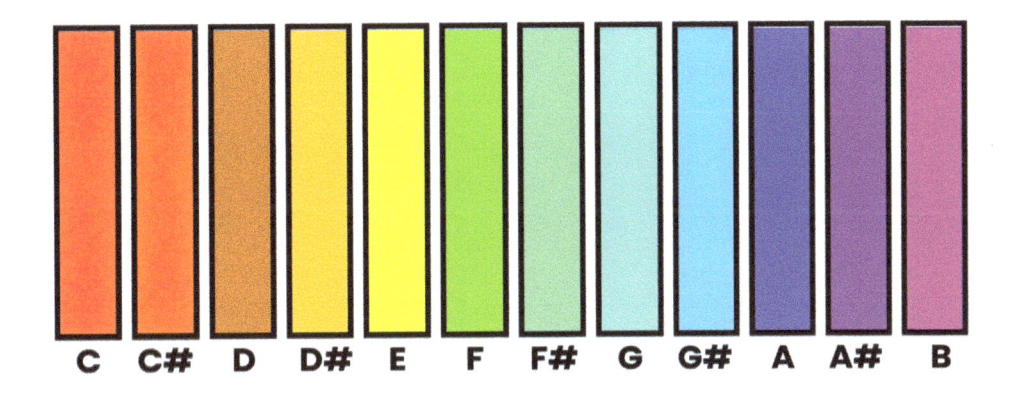

The above diagram shows musical notes with their corresponding colours

Colour

When white light is directed at a pyramid or prism the light is refracted and split into several different colours. This is known as the visible light spectrum. If we could listen to the colours they would make a note or tone because each colour vibrates at a different frequency.

The body is made up of seven major organs that vibrate at a certain frequency. The frequency that each organ vibrates on gives a tone or a note on the musical scale. If we could see music we would be able to see each note as a colour in the visible light spectrum. The colour seen by some people is called your aura and can spread to 12 feet outwards from the body. Colours represent the seven major organs in vibration, which manifest themselves as colour.

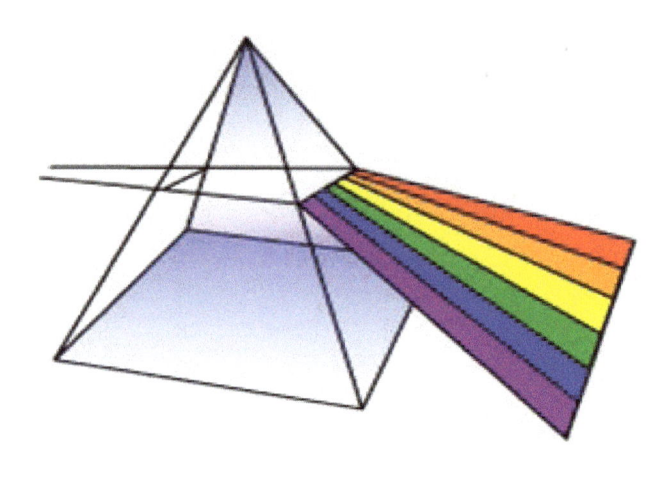

The above picture shows white light directed at a pyramid/prism

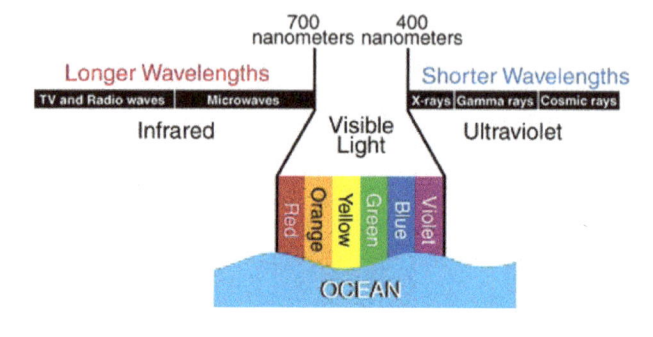

The above diagram shows the electromagnetic spectrum

DIVINATION OF THE BODY MEMBERS

PRT EM HRU
PLATE XXXII

My Hair is of NU

My Face is of RA

My two eyes are of HTHRU

My two ears are of APUAT

My nose is of KHENT-SHEPS

My two lips are of ANPU

My teeth are of KHEPERA

My neck is of AST

My two hands are of KHENEMU

My forearms are of NEITH

My Backbone is of SUT

My vagina is of MUT (females)/My phallus is of ASAR (males)

My thighs are of KHERABA

My chest is of SESEF-T-U

My belly and back are of SERKET

My buttocks are of the EYE of HRU

My hips and legs are of NUT

My feet are of PTAH

My fingers and toes are of the LIVING ARAT-U [Urei]

Not a member of mine is without Divinity

TEHUTI is protecting my flesh entirely

I AM RA every day... I come forth advancing

Seer of Millions of years is my name, travelling along the path of HRU

I feel... I perceive... I am in the UTCHAT... I exist by its Strength

I come forth and I shine... I go in and I come to life... My seat is on my throne

I sit in the pupil of my eye by it... I have commanded my seat

I rule it by my mouth speaking and in silence

I maintain an exact balance season from season

I Am, That I Am A Shining Being

Dwelling in (Black) Light, Dwelling in (Black) Light, Dwelling in (Black) Light

Dwelling in (Black) Light I Am.

Note: The words of a solar being.

Alternate Nostril Breathing – 'Utchat Nekhebet'

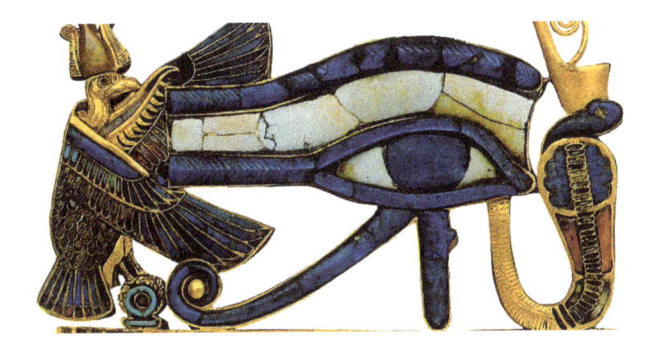

Smai Taui science has come to find, that 'Utchat Nekhebet' is very useful in stimulating the energy centres of the brain to produce clarity and clear the nervous system. It is useful for those who engage in a great deal of mental work, giving them a clear direction and allowing them to view their work with a refreshed mind. The exercise is also useful for those engaged in physical labour promoting a physical sense of wellbeing.

Sit erect in 'Nefertem' lotus or adept posture keeping the spinal column straight and the eyes in front. Let the hands rest on the upper part of the legs. Breathe with earth breath* (see page 89) breath rhythmically and steadily for a few moments. Begin Utchat Nekhebet breath by closing the left nostril with the right ring finger. Fold the index and pointing fingers down towards the fleshy part of your palm and press the right nostril close with the right thumb. Curl your tongue back to the roof of your mouth to stimulate the energy channel. You may find that your eyes roll back. If this naturally happens, let it, as you're connecting to the cerebral cortex of the brain. Remove the thumb from the right nostril and inhale through the right nostril. Then close with the thumb and release the right ring finger from the left nostril, and then exhale through the left nostril.

Without changing the fingers, inhale through the left, then close for a count of three. Then exhale through the right (to the count of nine) and inhale through the right (to the count of nine), and so on until this becomes a rhythmic cycle of breathing nine times from each nostril. Alternate nostrils as mentioned above, closing the unused nostril with the thumb or ring finger. This is one of the oldest forms of Smai breathing, and with visualization, it is a powerful tool of energy channel clearing.

1. Sitting in easy or *Nefertem* posture, cultivate nostril breathing nine times holding the breath for three counts. Work up to 19 times. Finish with HU.

2. Chant Aum Atum Aum Atun Aum Amun Aum nine times.

Visualize a brilliant white disc on the centre of your forehead – this represents the undifferentiated, the life centre. Chant Ankh nine times. Visualize a shining white cobra emerging from the left side of the disk – this is Utchat. Keep chanting and as you chant nine times, visualize a white shining cobra coming from the right side of the white disc – this is Nekhebet. Sit and feel the energy flowing through your median line in the spine, feel the flow of positive energy throughout the body and mind. This is usually practised for an entire month to detoxify the nervous system and beautify the body.

The entire meditation is around 15 mins. Sit for longer if you feel to do so.

Background information

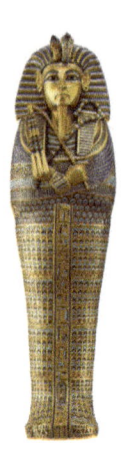

Utchat Cobra and Nekhebet *Vulture*, also known as Utchat and Udjat in Ancient Egypt, as the eye of Osiris/Asaru, the Sun and eye of Horus/Heru, the Moon, are sometimes depicted as two serpents on the crown of the Pharaoh lighthouse.

Alternate Nostril Breathing – 'Utchat Nekhebet' is known as a polarization exercise. In the Indian system, these two serpents are known as Pingala and Ida. The Nadis – *Indian*, Shabul – *Tama-rean/Kemetic* energy channels in the body.

Channels	KMT	Vedic	ANS
Solar	Utchat	Pingala	Sympathetic
Lunar	Nekhebet	Ida	Parasympathetic

Utchat/Solar Shabul channel is the right nostril which heats up the body. Used for physical activity and to help eliminate disease in the body. Utchat Lower Egypt – Per-Nu *'The Flame House' Cairo, Alexandria, etc.*

Nekhebet/Lunar Shabul channel is the left nostril that cools down the body. Used for calming and de-stressing. Nekhebet Upper Egypt – Per-Wer, 'The Great House', Esna, Aswan, Nubia, etc.

Alternate Nostril Breathing harmonizes both the solar and lunar channels, balancing (polarizing) the energy of the mind and body.

Nekhebet – Lunar Breath/ Northern Pole

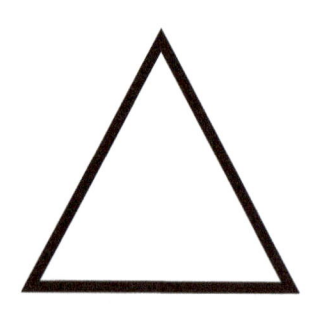

Protector of Upper Egypt, the south of the country

Ascending sacred triangle. Third Eye, Pineal Gland

Utchat – Solar Breath/ Southern Pole

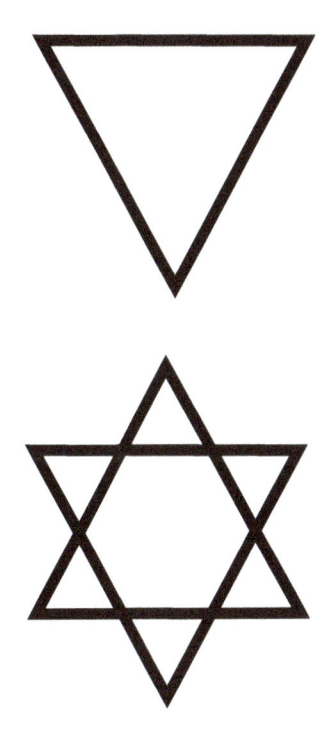

Protector of Lower Egypt, the north of the country

Descending sacred triangle.
Tonsils – Thyroid
Submental – Barathary gland

The 2 triangles are affected by the central tetrahedron, 'the Nose', through which the life force Sekhem is taken in to the body, giving Ankh-Life, Udja-Vitality, Seneb- Health

Unification of the Lighthouse – Brain hemispheres

Nekhebet	Utchat
Tefnut	Shu
Feminine Principle	Masculine Principle
Right Brain	Left Brain
Timeless	Time Bound
Asks Why?	Asks Why?
Processes info all at once	Processes info bit by bit
Simultaneous	Sequential
Looks at the whole	Looks at the detail
Connects the world	Splits the world into into a related whole
Looks for relationships	identifiable pieces
	Looks for causes and effects

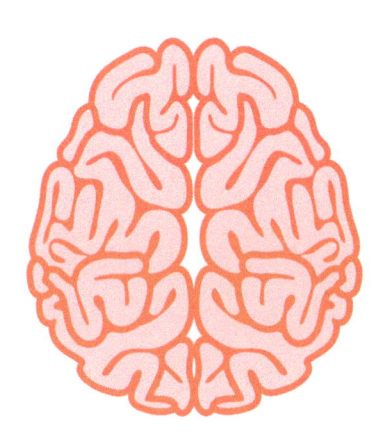

Focuses on emotions	Focuses on information
Uses pictures, shapes and colours	Uses words to name, describe and define
Inductive (going beyond the information given)	Deductive (all the information given is necessary for a conclusion and is contained in a premise)
Responds to words as images and	Tends to focus on grammar symbols
Can remember complex images	Remembers complex motor sequences

SMAI TAUI
Cosmic unity of complementary pairs

Tefnut/Cosmic Mother	Shu/Cosmic Father
Internal genitals	External genitals
Receptive	Perceptive
Cosmic Energy	Cosmic Consciousness
Individual Soul	Universal Soul
Nature	Spirit
Passive	Active
Lunar/cooling	Solar/warming
Left Nostril	Right Nostril
Right brain hemisphere	Left brain hemisphere
Para-sympathetic NS	Sympathetic NS
Magnetic	Electrical
Alkaline	Acidic
Retains Energy	Discharges Energy
Prefers cuddly sensuality	Prefers raw sex
Intuitive/Emotional	Rational/Logical
Practical, down to earth	Abstract, lost in thought
Geared to survival	Needs adventure

Elemental focus Earth

*Earth Breath – in and out of the nose – visualize the colour yellow.

Hika

Aum Atum Aum Atun Aum Amun 9 x

These are known as the three suns, and the Hika used is called 'the opening'.

From the upcoming Smai Meditation Book – 'Inner Spheres Outer Realities Vol. 1: A Practical Guide to Smai Taui Meditation' – by Pablo Imani ©

AFRIKAN YOGA AND ITS BENEFITS

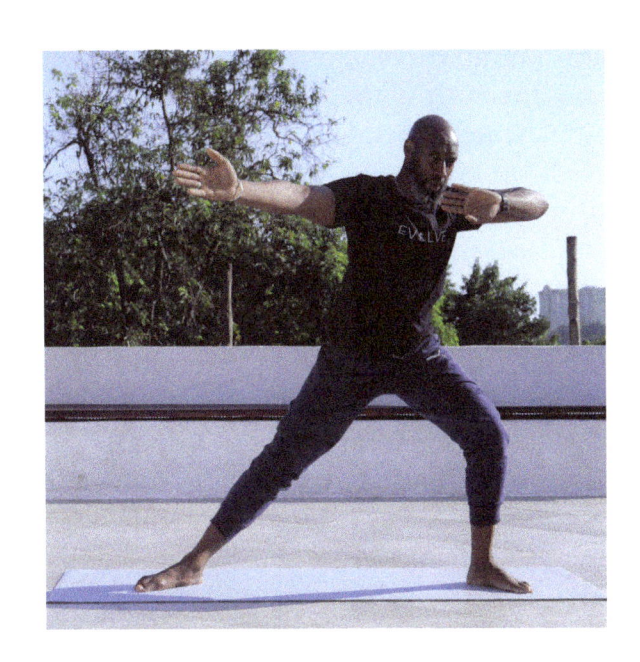

A PRAYER BEFORE A SESSION

The Prayer of Asar (Osiris):

I fly up from you, oh mortals!
I am not for the earth,
I am for the sky.
I have soared to the skies,
I have kissed the skies as a falcon,
I am the essence of deities,
The sun of deities,
The messenger of deities,
I am in the light of Re.
The light of Re is entering me,
I am life itself.

Warm-ups/Pa Raagus, the dance and Hudu (Afrikan Tai-chi)

This is the symbol for Aker. The combination of Tefnut and Shu that signifies the horizon, the point where night turns to day, where day turns to night. This is depicted as two lions seated back to back, facing away from each other. They are also called 'Yesterday and Tomorrow' as one lion faces towards the east, where the sun rises and begins the new day, the other lion faces west, where the sun sets and descends into the Underworld. They protect the western and the eastern horizons. Aker/Akiru also guards the gate to the Underworld and opens it for the King to pass through. According to a prominent Ancient Egyptian myth, the legendary 'gates of the afterworld' were guarded by two gigantic lions or sphinxes called Aker/Akiru. In New Kingdom tomb drawings, the Aker, sphinx of the eastern gate, sits proudly with its hind parts in a hollow. Underneath it, there can be seen a curious underground stream or duct. Behind the lion towers a huge mound or pyramid, and under it, a large oval chamber is found, which appears to be hermetically sealed.

Most of the warm-ups utilize ancient stretching techniques, which have been formed from Netert Tefnut 'moisture' and Shu 'air'; the two combined are known as HUDU (Afrikan Tai-Chi).

Egyptian Prayer

I acknowledge the four cardinal points of the universe:

The East, West, North and South.

I acknowledge the four elements of nature of which I am composed; there is no human or force lesser or greater than Earth, Water, Fire, Air.

I acknowledge and give thanks and praises to the nine planets: Earth, Jupiter, Mars, Mercury, Neptune, Pluto, Saturn, Uranus, Venus; to the stars, especially the Orion constellation Sirius A & B, to the sun and moon, and all cosmic entities.

I acknowledge all my ancestors (ask what you want).

May your vibrational force, invisible particles, positive transmissions enter into the nine openings in my body, through the pores of my skin, through the mole of my head.

Cleanse me of all negativity and bad vibrations and make me whole, pure as the breath of Shu, which circulates in all areas of my body.

May my words be pure.
May my heart be pure.
May my hands be pure.
Amun

Repeat 50x

AIR & WATER

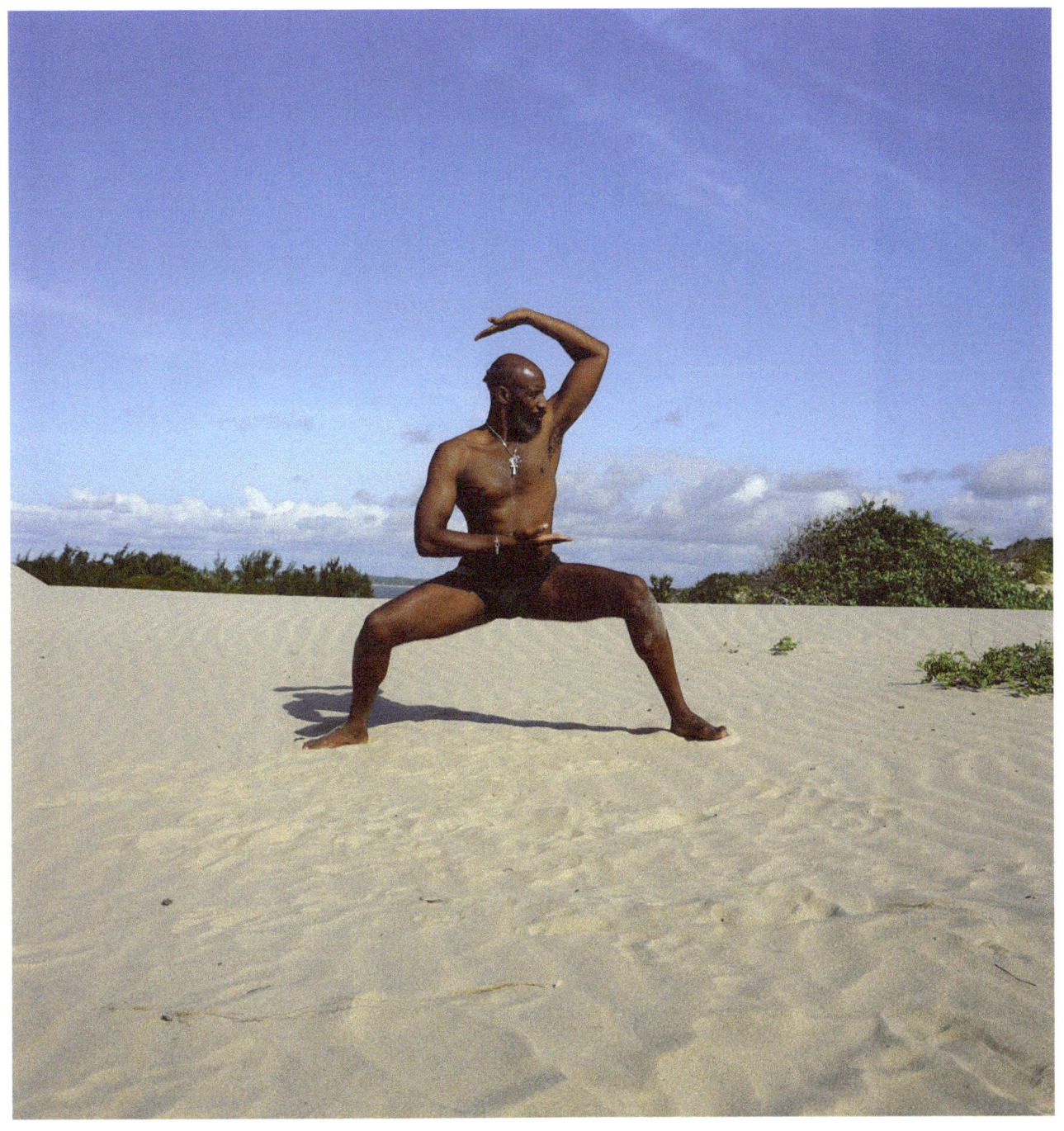

THE RE-EMERGENCE OF TAMA-RE SMAI TAUI AFRIKAN YOGA

Holding the Plates

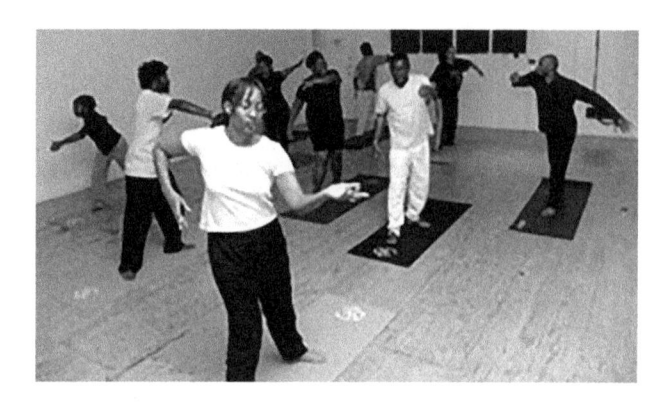

Holding the plates is a fun way of stretching utilizing breath, imagination and dance. Stand upright with legs shoulder-width apart. Turn your palms upwards keeping the fingers together and imagine that you are holding a plate on each hand with your dinner on it.

Begin to reach forward and outward slowly at first, guiding the plates around your body in sweeping movements, twisting your torso; inhale and exhaling deeply. Keep your palms facing upwards as the object is not to drop your plate.

You twist and turn your wrist in and out according to your movements; avoid turning your palms down or sideways so as not to drop your dinner.

Each stretch is precise and deliberate, yet you flow like a summer breeze. Use your imagination; the more experience you become, the more you can stretch the legs and use balancing techniques etc., speeding up as your confidence grows.

Plant and Harvest

This movement or hudu looks like the jinga in Capoeira and ngoma in Kazimba. The first phase of this hudu is to stand upright with the legs wide apart and outstretch one arm further than the other. Twist the body side to side throwing one arm behind you and as you twist around lean back.

Once you have done this a few times using deep breathing, begin to sweep the floor lightly with both hands, still twisting the torso in rhythmic movement, building momentum.

The second phase is to continue sweeping the floor and now to rise up after each sweep twisting the torso, leaning back and throwing your arms back over your shoulder. This is an enactment of an Afrikan story of planting and harvesting, where as you sweep, you are picking vegetation and placing it in the basket on your back.

This warms up and increases the flexibility of the spine and torso, and works the legs, ankles and knees. It develops concentration and rhythm.

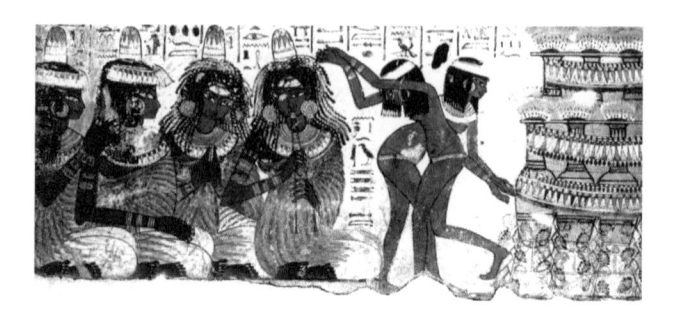

Pulling the Boat of Re

Stand with feet wide apart and imagine you are taking hold of a rope by turning to the side and stretching out an arm, pull and exhale. Inhale, and then stretch out the other arm to continue pulling the rope. Begin to do this with a continuous stream of rhythmic movement. Keep the legs wide as you lean to grab and bend the knee facing the imaginary rope, stretching the back leg. Change sides and pull there for a while;

without stopping the flow of movement, begin pulling from other directions above and below, and from behind.

Palm Tree

The palm tree utilizes side bends that stretch the torso, arms and hips, creating greater flexibility in those areas and releasing anxiety.

Stand upright with feet together. Place one hand behind your back and the other arm and hand pushed straight up. Let this arm rest alongside your ear. Inhale and lean towards the opposing side of the arm pushing straight up as far as you can, and exhale, and return to the position. Change arms and repeat the process.

The Practice

Guidance Notes:

1. Always warm up.
2. Never push yourself to the point of pain.
3. Always relax in between Sanuyaat/postures.
4. When in Sanuy, use the breath.
5. When in Sanuy, bear in mind the deity of the posture.

Yoga movements, in particular movements that are extreme positions, should be performed slowly. This is to ensure there is conscious control of the muscles; jerky or rapid movements are not controlled and can result in an injury.

All yoga movements start with a ready position. In this ready position preparatory breathing is carried out, which is inhalation and exhalation; this is an initiation process for the movement.

Injuries in the joints or muscles are most likely to occur when the muscles are out of control either through jerky movements, speed, lack of breath or the incorrect approach to the movement.

Note: *Sanuy* in Luganda, the language of the Muganda in Uganda of the Nile Valley, means *'happy'*. When you are performing and engaged in your posture, let it be a happy experience, take time, enjoy and create.

Pa Baagum Istamzaab 'The Standing Position'

The standing position lengthens the whole body and re-establishes the balance of the body. In the standing position stand tall, keep the head erect, look straight ahead; the back is kept straight, the feet are slightly apart and the arms are hanged loosely by the sides; that is considered to be the ideal position for a number of breathing techniques due to the fact that the distribution of muscular stress is fairly even throughout the entire body.

Breathe deeply into the abdomen and on the inhale push the stomach out. Exhale and draw the entire abdomen towards your spine.

Neck rolls

Humans carry a lot of tension in their necks, shoulders and upper back. Applying neck rolls before beginning Sanuyaat/postures will help release the tension and blocked energy trapped in the neck, shoulders and upper back. You may do this either sitting in easy pose or standing erect, where the body's weight is evenly distributed.

EYE OF RE AYUN SHIL USA

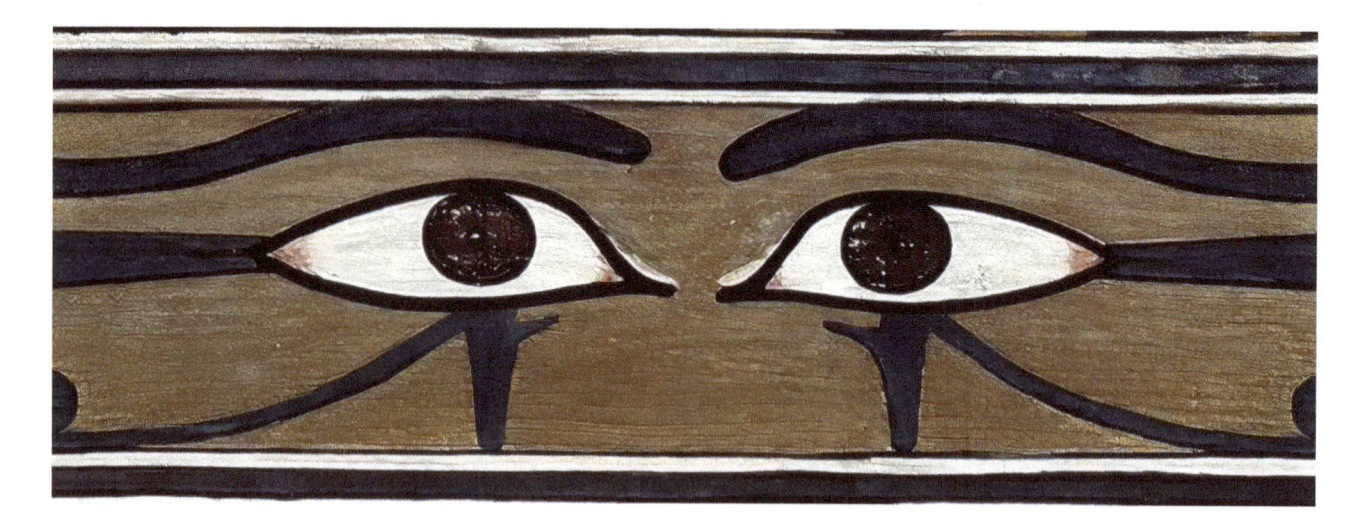

The Usa eye of Re is known as 'the all-seeing eye'. However, this eye is commonly referred to as 'the third eye', the spiritual eye that perceives; views things, events and happenings in different dimensions and time. It is, in reality, the first eye. All-seeing and all-knowing, this eye is the eye we possess, linked to our divinity, especially, at birth. When a newborn arrives, his or her third eye is open. If born in a hospital, the doctors and nurses shine bright artificial light on the mother and child. These bright lights are a shock to a newborn, who has grown in a darkened womb, accustomed to seeing in the dark and perceiving things through touch, vibration and his/her third eye. The artificial light immediately causes an adverse effect on the child, and the third eye begins to shut down, and has to be reactivated through a DNA explosion. That is why in Ancient Afrikan culture, we keep the child in a darkened room for days – sometimes 10 days – until the child grows more accustomed to its new environment, where there is night and day, and the third eye more or less remains intact.

In KMT the eyes are important symbols of Re, Asar and Heru: in combination, their power to see all is unlimited. The eye of Asaru is known as the Utchat – this represents the sun; and the eye of Heru is the Udjat, which is a night eye/shadow or moon. Many confuse these eyes and are unaware that they are three with interchangeable attributes; and many often refer to this eye as the 'evil eye', ignorant to the fact that the eye itself is not evil, but the eye witnesses evil.

There are those who fear these eyes and teach the fear of them because they feel they are unable to do wickedness in the presence of the eye of Re as they will be seen and revealed. These eyes are superimposed on the brow arush and pineal gland. Heru was gifted the eye of Re when he lost one of his eyes in the battle with Set, and this is why the eye of Heru is often referred to as 'the eye of Ra/Re'.

"The pupil is the black dot, the portal through which light passes through the black doorway of the collective consciousness. Blackness appears to be darkness (ignorance) to a Sethian lower mind consciousness. It evokes fear of the dense material matter that cannot be penetrated by a strictly logical mind. BLACKNESS or the VEIL OF ISIS (consciousness) does invite communication by the way of the heart, highly evolved feeling, tone and intuition. It is this faculty of feeling, tone, intuitive mind that is the hallmark of the Afrikan mind, immersed in symbolism and fluent in the language of time and space."

Dr Richard King MD, *African Origin of Biological Psychiatry*

Eye exercises

The eye is brain tissue and links in with cognitive workings of the brain through the various nerve cells known as reticular formation. The exercise of the eyes assists the brain to be alert and balanced in the left and right hemispheres.

"Do not despise the body for it is the temple of the living spirit."

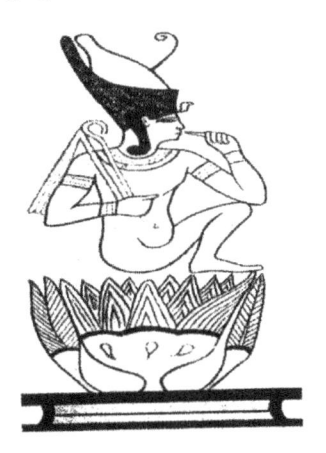

Sitting Sanuyaat for meditation

All of the various sitting positions for meditation are calming and nurturing; some promote the opening of the hips and require more effort. In general, when practised properly with the spine and pelvis aligned, they endorse a great deal of vitality, improving the circulation, reducing fatigue, soothing the nervous system and centering the mind.

These positions of meditation can be done at any time; however, the best time is in the morning after a yoga practice, when the body is warm and the limbs loose. Sitting will be easier and more welcoming as the mind will be focused and less cluttered with the day's work. The positions are a recommended daily practice alongside your Afrikan Yoga/Smai Sanuyaat practice.

While in these positions, you can also choose any 'Taruh' hand position you wish or naturally require. (Please refer to Taruh Hand positions on page 122.) You can use a pillow, cushion or folded blanket to sit on for comfort.

Pa Jaalus Istamzaab or The sitting Heru/Hero

The Sitting Heru Sanuy or position is one form that most of us will be familiar with, especially if you have been taught to pray or prostrate as a child, as it involves kneeling and being still. This is also part of the final sequence of the Ashutat prayer positions and movements of the Egyptians. This position is known to Indian Yogis as 'The Rock'. The word 'hero' comes from Heru or which the Greeks named Horus, the falcon deity and the legendary hero of Ancient Egypt.

From Horus we also derived the words: horizon, horizontal, hours and horoscope. Before attempting this, make sure you can sit comfortably in this position for more than a minute. Make sure the heels are pointed straight up for correct alignment and knee protection.

Start by kneeling on the floor with your buttocks comfortably on the back of your legs. Feel your feet open to support your buttocks and slightly lift the knee to release tension from the knee caps. Make the spine tall and place the hands on top of the thighs, bringing them slightly apart. Move the pelvis forward; sit for nine deep breaths.

For advanced Heru, your buttocks touch the floor with your feet folded straight back along your thighs. Breathe deeply into your abdomen for nine breaths.

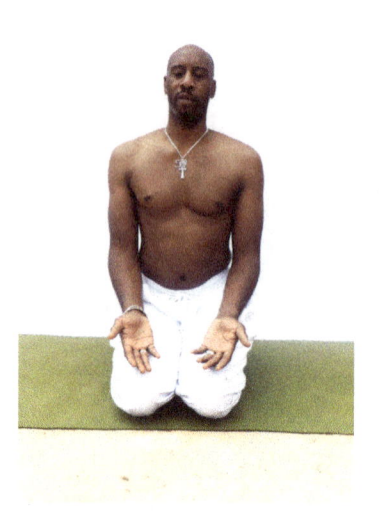

Easy Pose

This is for developing a positive and steady base for the body, and keeping the energy centred. When sitting in this pose, you can use a hand taruh, the ancient positions of thumb and index or any other finger, or clasping the hands together in an interlocking position (Aset). Another alternative is placing the hands in your lap, one hand in the other. Easy pose calms the mind and relaxes the body in preparation for meditation. The position assists the opening of the hips and is a comfortable sitting position for meditation and breathing exercises.

Begin by sitting on the mat cross-legged. Allow your feet to rest below the knees.

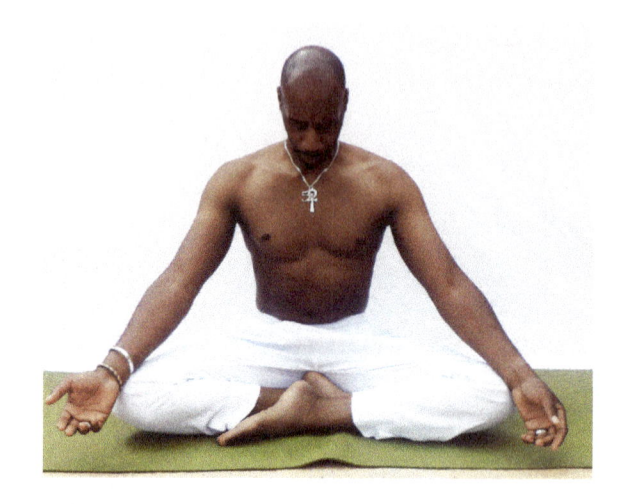

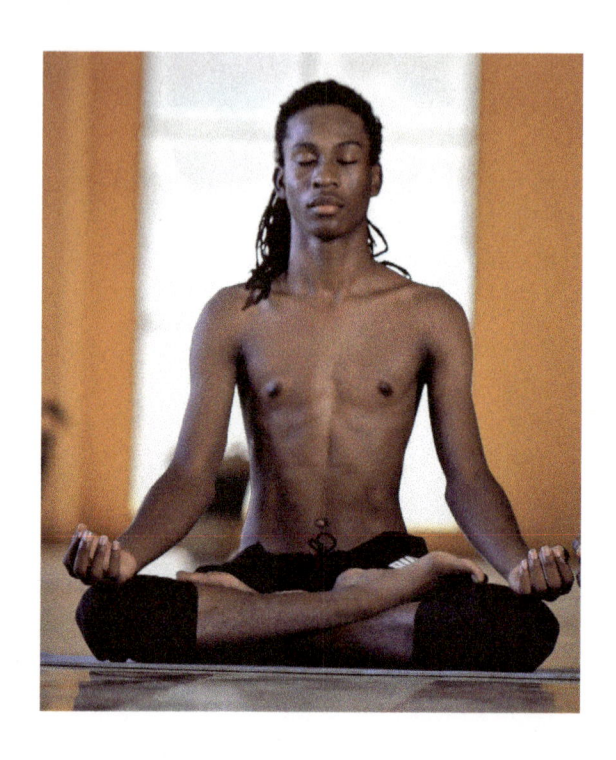

Nefertem 'Beautiful Completion' (full Lotus)

The lotus position is probably the most recognizable posture of yoga. From Buddha and Buddhism to Mystics and Sufism, to Bruce Lee in the movie 'Enter the Dragon', this posture is renowned the world over for centring and focusing the mind.

There is a prayer or request you can use in Nefertem for being transformed into the lotus taken from *'Coming Forth by Day'* Translated by Amunnubi Ruakh Ptah:

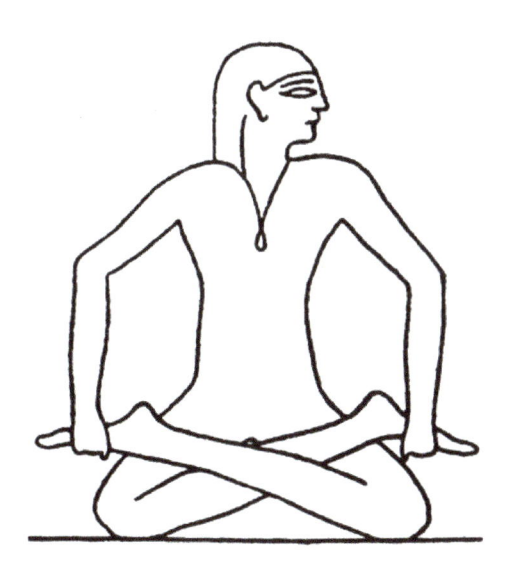

Kemetic Lotus

1. O Lotus,
2. Belonging to the semblance of Nefertum, 'The perfectly Beautiful',
3. I am the Man,
4. I know your names, you, Neteru,
5. You, the Masters of the Neter's Domain,
6. For I am one of you.
7. May you grant that I see the Neter's Domain, in the presence of the Masters of the West.
8. May I take my place that it desires.
9. Without being held back from the presence of the Great Ennead (Nine Neteru).

Note: Inhale deeply and lengthen your spine drawing your shoulders back, allowing the shoulder blades to gently slide closer, relaxing the shoulders. Exhale and allow yourself to be rooted from your pelvic floor, gently softening into the pose. Relax, breathing steadily and rhythmically. Sit as long as you wish.

You may also use a Hikau of Yaa Nefertem 24 times in the morning to develop youthfulness, enthusiasm and vigour.

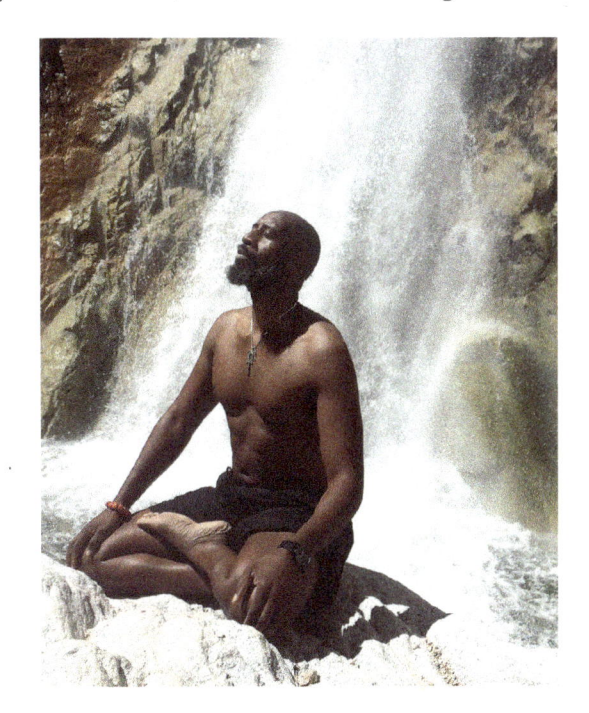

Nefertem rising (Half Lotus or Adept posture)

THE RE-EMERGENCE OF TAMA-RE SMAI TAUI AFRIKAN YOGA | 98

This Sanuy is close to Nefertum (full Lotus) and is often called the Easy pose as it does not require both feet to be high on the thigh.

Sit with your legs extended in front of you, and make your spine tall by sitting up. Draw one heel towards your navel and turn your foot and leg outward, and place it on your lap at the top of your thigh. Draw your other heel towards your navel and turn the foot and leg outward placing them on the top of your opposite thigh.

Wrap your toes over your thighs flexing and pressing them down into your thighs.

Widen your thighs and keep the spine tall by sitting up.

Draw one heel towards your navel and turn your foot and leg outward, and place it on your lap at the top of your thigh. Alternatively, you can place one foot on top of the lower calf. Inhale deeply and lengthen your spine drawing your shoulders back, allowing the shoulder blades to gently slide closer, relaxing the shoulders. Exhale and allow yourself to be rooted from your pelvic floor, gently softening into the pose. Relax, breathing steadily and rhythmically.

The benefits are:

Physically

1. It opens the hips
2. Increases knee flexibility and lubricates the knee joints
3. Prevents arthritis and osteoporosis
4. Tones the abdominal and encourages digestive functions

Mentally

1. Nefertem focuses the mind
2. Reduces stress and brings mental clarity

Contraindications

Do not use this pose if you have low back, knee or hip injuries.

Nun (The primordial waters/collective unconsciousness)

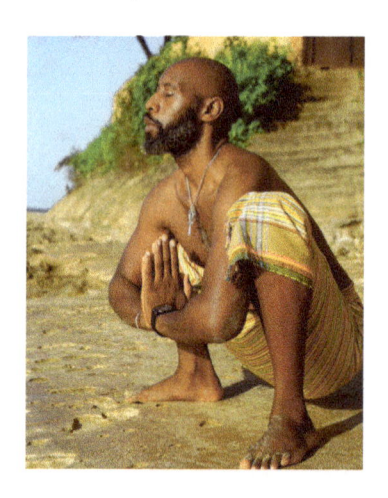

Nun relates to (the mythological) primordial waters or (the cosmic) boundless universe, which is the macrocosm of the womb in the physical realm. This is why Sanuy Nun is seen when Afrikan women give birth. Sanuy Nun is perfect for women in pregnancy. Afrikan women have been giving birth in this position for thousands of years.

This tends to be a natural position as gravity allows the baby to easily be born, whereas lying on your back with your legs up goes against gravity. This is a Greek invention used today in hospitals – it creates struggle, distress and bonding disruption. The position of Nun, especially in the last weeks of pregnancy to the latter part of the 3rd trimester, assists the baby to move into the correct position for labour. If the baby is in a breech position or you have cervical suture, do not perform Sanuy Nun. The posture is not recommended if you are also enduring painful haemorrhoids and varicose veins.

Begin by standing and place palms together in taful (prayer taruh) in front of your chest, bring the body down into a squat position keeping the back straight.

Keep your knees bending over your toes and use your elbows to open your knees, and stretch out the pelvis and hips. Straighten your spine as much as you can as you will be leaning forward. Hold comfortably for nine breaths.

The benefits of Sanuy Nun are:

1. The stretching of the pelvic region and raising a healthy blood supply to this region through the breath
2. Increases circulation
3. Releases premenstrual tension
4. Helps to release tension, eases aches and pains
5. Boosts fertility
6. Tones the inner thigh and abdominals
7. Strengthens the knees, bones and ligaments in the legs
8. Develops balance

In Sanuy Nun you can also perform *Hikau* (mantra) YAANUN 46 times for vitality.

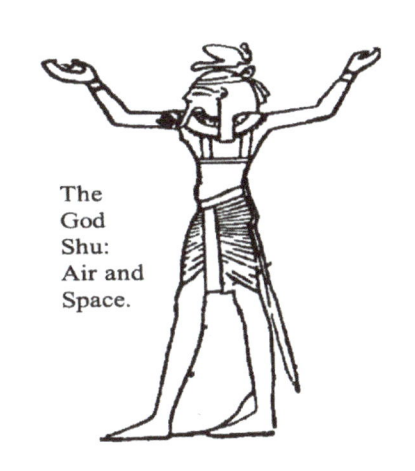

The God Shu: Air and Space.

SHU Pa Raafur Istamzaab 'The Raising Position'

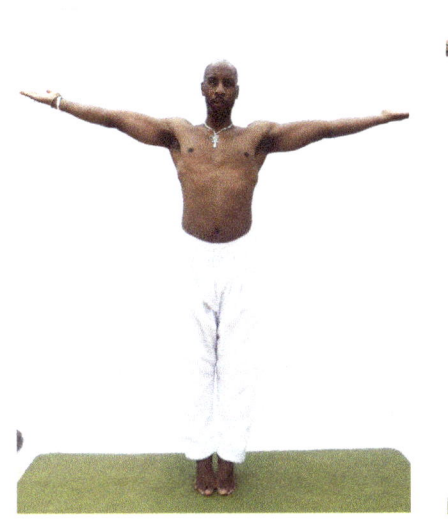

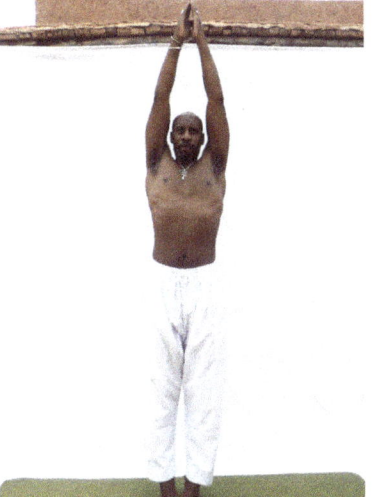

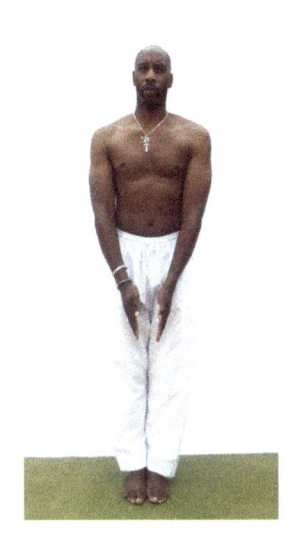

SHU is often called the 'complete breathing technique' by some yogis. For Complete Breath, the arms are raised slowly sideways and upwards. During breath retention in this exercise, the arms should be overhead.

When performing the complete breath, the diaphragm undergoes expansion allowing for brief dislodgement of internal abdominal organs to experience a massage and to gently be relocated during exhalation.

This breathing technique improves the co-ordination of several systems of the body and incorporates all three: diaphragm, intercostal and clavicle breathing. This is where the expansion of the diaphragm, ribs, sternum and lungs comes into play by steady, slow and continuous inhalation of air through the nose; and an equal exhalation occurs to expel the air with the sound YAASHUUUUUUU.

SHU also adds to the legs, calves and toe muscles by toning them as you rise on your toes. Shu develops your sense of balance and self-trust.

Use hikau Yaa Shu 38 times to draw the healing forces of Sekhem throughout your being through each breath.

Earth
Katuf Bagum: Shoulder Stand or
'Pa Banur': The Candle

Katuf Bagum or Candle will have a wonderful effect on the body as it stimulates the thyroid and opens the sekhemic flow of energy in the internal organs via the ley lines of the body known as meridians.

Begin by lying on your back in a supine position, hands at the sides of the body, palms on the floor. Bring the chin in towards the chest – this assists the movement. The spinal column must be as flat as possible.

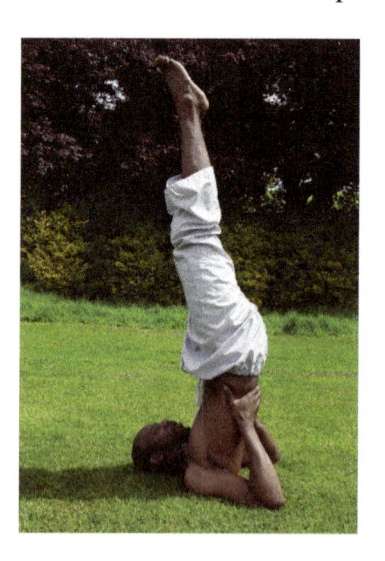

If beginners are unable to keep their backs flat, they may start with their knees bent. The legs are raised slowly and together in one continuous movement with grace and deliberateness until they reach a vertical position.

Begin to raise the buttocks and push the legs up vertically and raising the entire torso up, balancing on the shoulders, supporting your back with your hands.

Keep your hands on your back by the kidneys with your fingers turning towards the spinal centre and adjust as you see fit. Align the body focusing on perfection and the straightness of a candle. Bring the elbows in and slightly more close together.

The benefits of Katuf Bagum are:

1. Stimulates the thyroid gland
2. Stretches the spinal column
3. Massages the heart, lungs
4. Encourages good circulation of the blood
5. Prevents sluggishness

6. Assists in the relief of depression and poor sleeping patterns
7. Opens the flow of sekhemic energy in the internal organs, kidneys, small stomach, and gall bladder

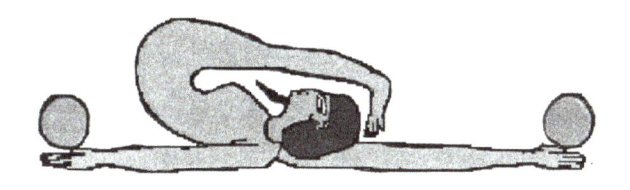

Geb: The Plough

This Sanuy is powerful as it works the entire spine, which contains the spinal cord, influencing the sympathetic nervous system.

The thyroid gland also benefits from Geb with an increase of fresh blood supply flowing to the area of the neck, throat and head.

This gland controls the metabolism and stimulates the youthfulness of the body. When not functioning at its optimum level, the body's skin becomes wrinkled and dry. Blood pressure and low sexual activity decreases with physical and mental laziness in tow.

The thyroid is the gland most likely to cause overweight and underweight in people as under-activity of this gland causes the release of hormones to be insufficient, which impedes physical and mental growth in children. Over-activity of the thyroid gland shows the exact opposite, causing increases in height, underweight, excitability and nervousness.

In adults, the overactivity of the gland may cause some of the same conditions: he/she may lose weight and become irritable, with a rapid pulse rate. Eyes also tend to bulge and glaze.

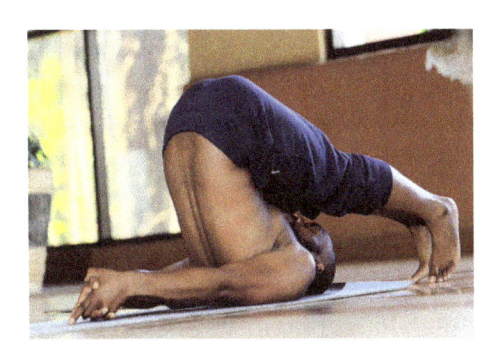

Begin by lying on your back in supine position, hands at the sides of the body, palms on the floor. Bring the chin in towards the chest – this assists the movement. The spinal column must be as flat as possible.

If beginners are unable to keep their backs flat, they may start with their knees bent. The legs are raised slowly and together in one continuous movement with grace and deliberateness until they reach a vertical position.

Begin to raise the buttocks and push the legs up vertically and raising the entire torso up, balancing on the shoulders, supporting your back with your hands.

Now that you are in the candle position, lower your legs over and away from your head. Allow the toes to touch the floor. Deepening the stretch, point the toes in towards the head. If your feet do not touch the floor at first, with practice your spine will lengthen, and your weight will eventually bear down. Always be relaxed and patient, allow for no jerky movements as the practice of Smai is graceful in all its aspects, and any jerks will be detrimental to your well-being. This completes the stretch acting on all regions of the vertebrae. Raise the legs and move back into Pa Banur (the candle), and slowly bend the knees toward the head, place the hands on the mat palms facing down and unravel the spine, dropping the body and legs towards the floor back into a supine position. Keep the back of the head firmly on the ground again avoiding any jerky movements.

Lie in mummy and relax.

The benefits of this Sanuy include:

Physically

1. Brings balance to the thyroid
2. Calms the nerves; it is very reviving and is useful for tiredness
3. Sends fresh blood flow towards the head, the brain and the face hence preventing wrinkles and lines
4. This movement is beneficial to the spleen and the sexual glands
5. The Sanuy Geb also stimulates the liver, assisting decongestion and cleansing, massaging the pancreas and kidneys
6. Useful for diabetics due to its effect on the pancreas
7. Works against constipation
8. Is effective against cellulitis and obesity by improving the function of the colon

Mentally

1. Enhances good posture and inner balance
2. Relieves insomnia and restless sleep

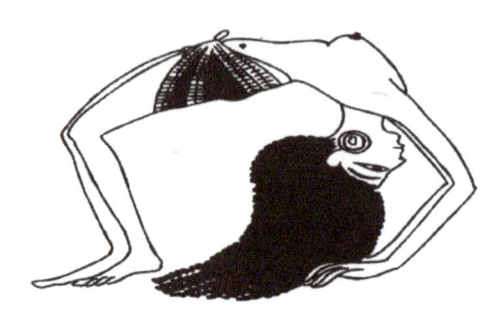

Kemetic Wheel

Shen: The Wheel

Begin in the supine position of lying on your back, legs outstretched, palms by your side facing up. Bend your knees and bring your heels towards your buttocks. Keep your feet hip-width apart and flat on the floor. Bend the arms backwards and place your palms just above the shoulders with the fingers directed towards your feet.

Inhale. Raise your pelvis and hips upwards, then press your fingers into the floor and push upwards keeping your feet rooted to the floor. Your shoulder blades will draw inwards and into your back – allow this as long as the shoulders do not tighten up. If the shoulders do tighten, widen them a bit by bringing the arms out. Spread your fingers and push further into an arch forming the SHEN, hold for several breaths. Bend the elbows and draw the head in towards the chest while lowering yourself onto your back and exiting the Sanuy.

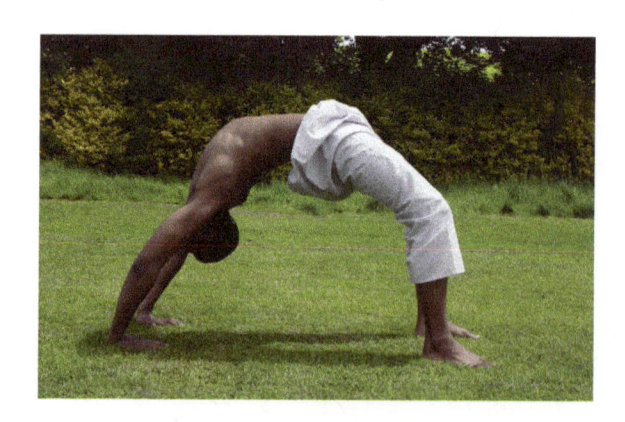

The benefits of this Sanuy include:

Physically

1. The entire spine maintaining its strength and suppleness
2. The strengthening of the thighs and hips
3. The wrists, forearms, shoulders and spine – all receive a stretch
4. Opens up the chest cavity increasing the lung capacity
5. The movement also strengthens and tones the buttocks, legs, chest, back shoulders and wrists
6. Stimulates the lymph, reproductive and digestive systems
7. Assists in infertility, osteoporosis, backache, and asthma
8. Stimulates the thyroid and pituitary gland
9. Helps to increase your stamina

Mentally

1. Energizes the mind
2. Relieves mild depression
3. Relieves anxiety and reduces stress

Contraindications

Do not do this movement if you have high or low blood pressure, back and knee or neck injury, or carpal tunnel syndrome.

Manjet 'The Boat of Re'

The Manjet is a semi inverted Sanuy. It entails more of a backward bend and is viewed as a counterpose to the Katuf Bagum Sanuy alongside the Shen Sanuy.

Begin by lying flat on your back and place your palms under your thighs, turn the palms upwards, breathing gently and regularly. Keep the legs straight and point the toes upwards, and the heels down into the floor. Raise your body upwards turning the shoulder blades in and pressing down on to the elbows as the upper body is raised off the ground. The legs remain straight and on the ground. Balance your weight on your elbows, arch the back and drop your head backwards, lowering the body on top of the head. It is important that you keep the weight on the elbows, as your head only touches the ground slightly. Now breathe a little more deeply but maintain a regular breath. Allow the chest to open up further and keep the shoulder blades together. You may gaze directly behind you on a certain spot or object if you need to focus.

When finished, press down on the elbows and lift the head off the ground and back into a tilt position before lowering the head. Now just allow the body to drop gently back down on to the mat in mummy Sanuy.

The benefits of this Sanuy include:

1. The stretching of the intestines and abdominals
2. It promotes deep breathing and assists in the alleviation of backache
3. The pelvis is also stretched
4. The shoulders and arms are strengthened and toned

5. The thyroid, thymus and pineal glands are stimulated
6. Focus is on the solar plexus

Geb/Spinal Twist

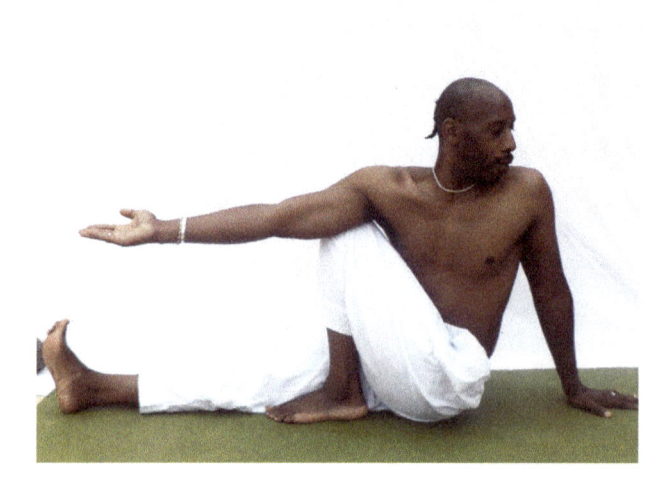

This Sanuy is another wonderful posture that works the entire spine.

Begin by sitting on the mat, legs outstretched in front of you, feet together. Bend or double up the right leg and bring your feet alongside your left knee, let the anklebone touch the outside of the knee. The right foot is flat on the ground and parallel with the left leg. Now place the right arm back and lean back slightly (only a touch) with the right hand flat on the floor, fingers spread wide apart. Allow the hand to take your weight. Now draw your body up towards your thigh, as your back should be upright as much as possible. Place your left arm across your torso and lever it around the right knee making it parallel with the outstretched left leg. Now with this outstretched arm, turn the palm facing upwards.

The left arm is inducing the shoulders to turn and therefore create the twist in the spine without offering any resistance. The head now turns looking over the right shoulder at the same time stretching the neck, completing 'Geb spinal twist'. Hold for nine breaths.

The Sanuy is also practised on the other leg, where the left leg is bent, and the left arm and hand are placed on the floor, etc.

Concentrate on the relaxation of the spinal structure and the shoulders and follow mentally the twist from the sacrum up to the skull.

The benefits of this Sanuy include:

1. Stretches and lengthens the spine and all the muscles and ligaments in the spinal vertebrae
2. Tones up the muscles in the back through the rush of blood flow
3. Tones up the entire organism of the body as it works the nerves of the spinal cord
4. Stimulates and has a great effect on the nervous system, commonly called the immune system, which is strengthened by the spinal twist
5. Increases the flexibility of the spine
6. Removes and relieves muscular problems in the back
7. Massages the abdominals
8. Positive effects on the spleen, gall bladder, kidneys, liver, and bowels
9. Develops the sekhemic energy
10. Promotes peace of mind and stability

Sitting Nut/Forward Bend

Sit with legs extended. Inhale and press your hands down into the floor to lengthen your spine, bring your lower back in and upward making the back tall.

Inhale and bring your arms overhead. Exhale, bend forward and grasp your toes or alternatively grasp your big toes with your index and middle fingers.

Inhale and extend your belly up through to the top of your head. Tilt your pelvis forward and draw your lower back in. Anchor your thighs down and exhale widening your elbows out, and draw your torso forward towards your feet. Keep the legs engaged and straight. Bend the waist like a hinge and lead with the heart, bring the head forward moving towards the feet.

Repeat this stretch three times and hold each time for nine breaths – 19 for the more advanced.

The benefits of this Sanuy include:

1. Stretches the spine, hamstrings, and calves
2. Improves digestion
3. Stimulates the lymph and reproductive systems
4. Helps relieve menstrual, and menopause discomfort
5. Improves liver, kidney, and colon function
6. Massages the abdominal organs
7. Increases elasticity in the joints
8. Alleviates high blood pressure and infertility
9. Keeps you youthful
10. Reduces fatigue and insomnia
11. Soothes the nervous system
12. Relieves stress, anxiety, and mild depression
13. Develops concentration and Sekhem energy
14. Assists in meditation

Contraindications

Lower back injury, asthma.
In pregnancy (use variations).

Mental Transformation Sanuyaat

Selket Scorpion

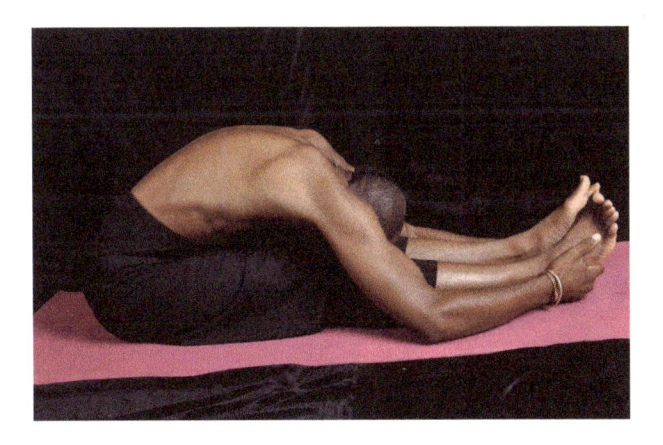

The movement of the legs in Selket utilizes the muscles of the entire lower back strengthening the muscles of the lower back.

The practitioner lays flat on their stomach with the forehead placed down on to the mat. The legs are close together (at a beginner's level), the hands are made into a fist and tucked under the thighs. Alternatively, the hands and arms are stretched out forward and above the head. Palms are placed facing down just under the thighs.

It is very important that advanced or beginners start by using what is termed 'half scorpion', where one leg is raised on inhale – raise the leg as far as it can go keeping the leg straight and hold; lower the leg on the exhale.

Relax by turning the head onto its side. Repeat the movement on the opposing leg. Then raise both legs together using the same process of inhaling and lowering on exhale. The length of time you hold the breath can vary between three breaths up to nine breaths, however, it is important not to exceed nine breaths.

The benefits of this Sanuy include:

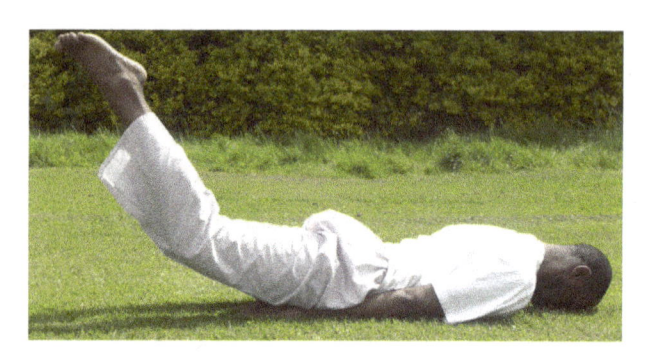

1. Utilizes the muscles of the entire lower back
2. The muscles of the lower back are strengthened considerably
3. Increases the flexibility of the back
4. Tones the lumbar and sacral region and is quite simple so anyone can perform it
5. Works and stimulates the kidneys
6. Stimulates the nervous system
7. Stimulates the solar plexus

Wadjet/UREAUS Cobra

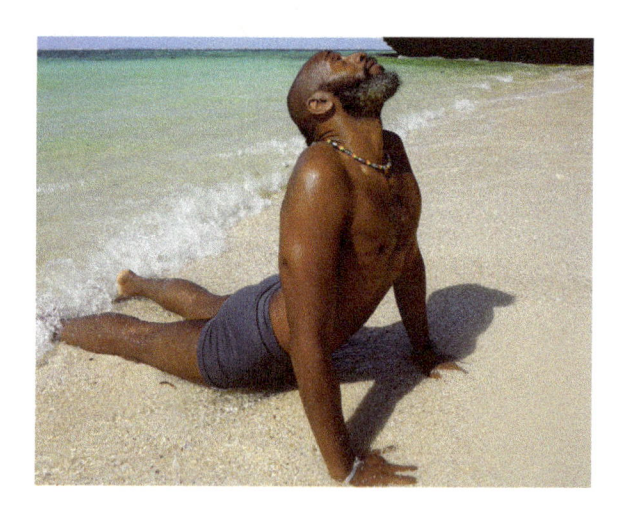

In supine position place hands palms down just under your shoulders. Keep the elbows on the ground and close to your sides. Turn the toes in and inhale. Raise the chest off the floor pushing upwards, using your hands and spreading your fingers whilst arching the torso up in the slow graceful movement of the cobra. Concentrate on the third eye and turn your toes out. Inhale and exhale holding as long as possible, keeping the shoulders relaxed. Repeat for as long as possible.

The benefits of this Sanuy include:

Physically

1. Massages the muscles in the back
2. Increases the spine flexibility
3. Expands the rib cage
4. Brings relief from asthma
5. Gently massages internal organs
6. Assists in the relief of numerous menstrual problems

Mentally

1. Develops the faculty of concentration
2. Releases Sekhem energy helping you realize your full potential

Sebek Crocodile

Start in a Dub/Scarab child position. Place both arms in front of you on the floor keeping them wide and bent at the elbows, making the form of a KA.

Draw the left leg back keeping the right knee bent.

Remain sitting slightly on your heel and inhale, and raise your head and chest, and arms off the floor stretching and arching the spine. Once you are balanced, exhale and gently settle back down to the floor, keeping the arms in the same position of a KA.

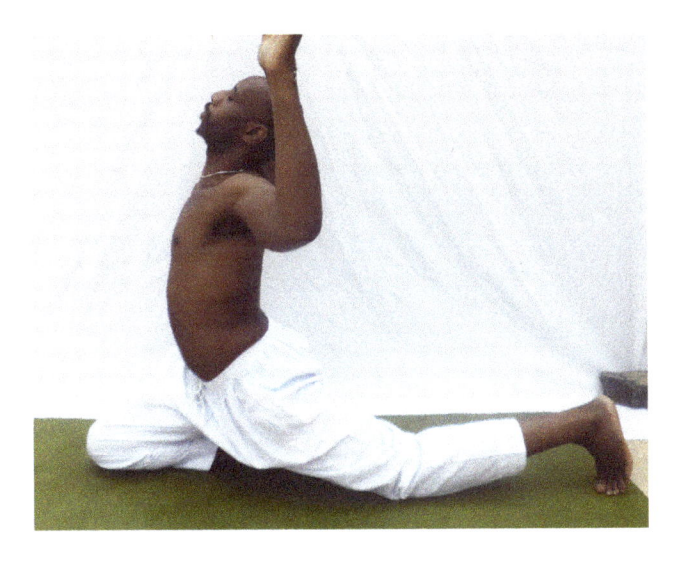

Draw the left leg back into a kneeling position of the Scarab. Repeat drawing the right leg back.

The benefits of this Sanuy include:

1. Stretches the hips and thighs
2. Stretches the spine
3. Opens the chest
4. Develops flexibility in the hips and back
5. Strengthens toes and ankles

FIRE

Pa Bast/ the Cat

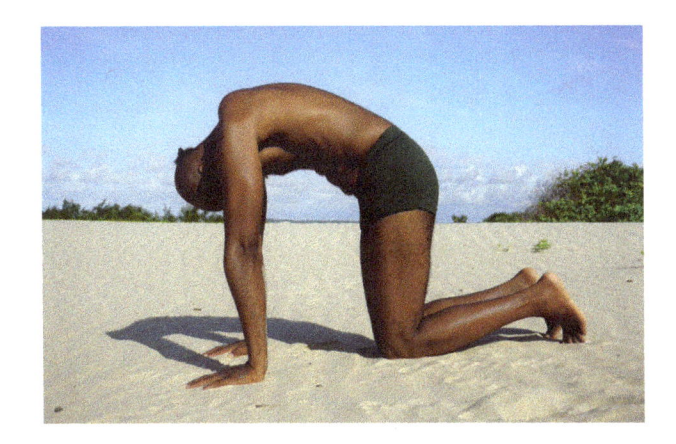

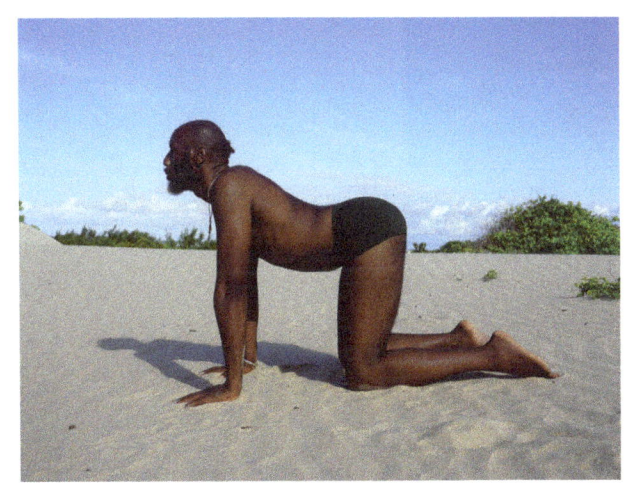

This Sanuy opens the back and stretches the spine and is beneficial for menstrual problems, delivering a flow of blood to the nervous system through the spine. Begin on all fours with your hands in line with your shoulders, and your knees and legs parallel but slightly apart. Inhale and raise the entire back arched upwards into a hump, stretching the shoulder blades. Bending the head inwards, rest the chin on the collarbone, looking towards the chest. Exhale and slowly lift the head, and at the same time drop the abdominals down towards the mat, and curve the back inwards.

Approaching the Higher Self

Standing Nut/Forward Bend

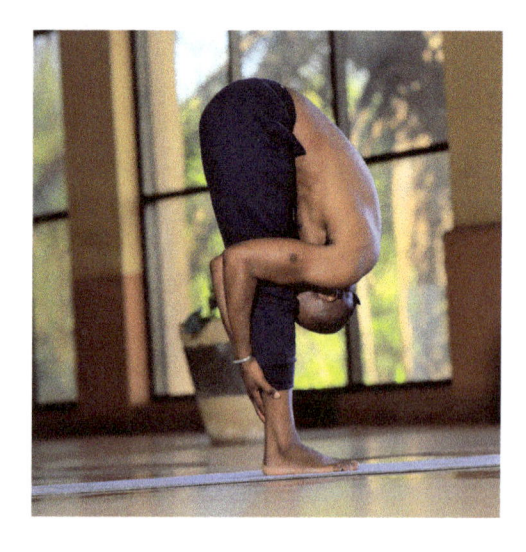

Begin by standing with your feet parallel, spread your toes and root yourself right down through all four corners of your feet. Inhale and raise your arms out to the side or push the arms up from the centre of your body. Extending your lower torso, push up through your fingertips. Maintain the length.

Exhale and bend forward reaching for your toes or the floor. Hold for a few breaths.

The benefits of this Sanuy include:

Physically

1. Lengthens the spine
2. Develops suppleness and elasticity
3. Mobilizes joints
4. Rejuvenates the nervous system
5. Stretches the hamstrings and muscles of the back of the leg
6. Increases blood supply to the brain
7. Burns off calories

Mentally

1. Gently enhances concentration
2. Dissolves laziness
3. Stimulates intelligent capacities

Heru/Haru

Heru/Haru Sanuy in the Indian system of yoga is called 'the mountain posture'; this is interesting as Har means 'on high'.

Begin by standing with feet slightly apart and shoulders relaxed, and hands down by your sides turning your palms facing forwards. Feel your weight evenly distributed on both feet and root yourself in the ground. Raise your head up so the neck and spine are stretched upward as if pulled by a thin thread. Lift your chest and breathe deeply and evenly pushing out the stomach on the inhale and bringing the stomach back towards the spine on the exhale. Listen to the sound of your breath and continue up to nine times. There should be no tension in you.

The meditation is on Heru who has conquered the lower natures.

The benefits of this Sanuy include:

Physically

1. Aligns the body posture
2. Assists in the distribution of weight evenly in the body
3. Improves balance

Mentally

1. Relieves mental tension
2. Promotes calm and self-assurance

Henu (Anpu, Heru, Set)

Standing Position

From Heru you move into Anpu, also known as Anubis. This Sanuy is known as a 'warrior pose' and is used in the form of tension dynamics.

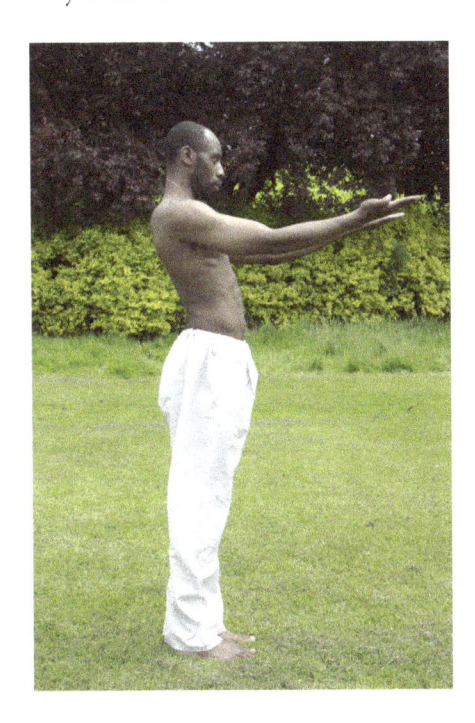

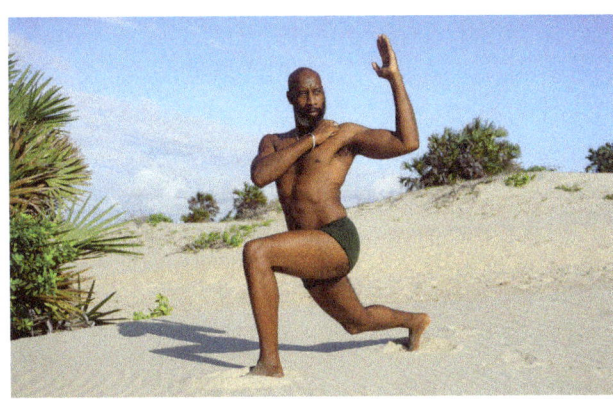

Begin by standing in Heru, then bend the elbow at an angle of 45 degrees. Raise both hands up directly in front of you, palms facing upwards, fingers together, and thumbs in. Then draw the left leg back, bending the knee and lowering it to the ground (advanced students do not touch the floor). Bring the arm of the bent leg across to the right shoulder curling the hand into a fist and bring the outstretched arm around to the side of the shoulder, bending the elbow, palm facing forward. Hold for four breaths and increase to nine breaths. Repeat on the other side of the body.

The benefits of this Sanuy include:

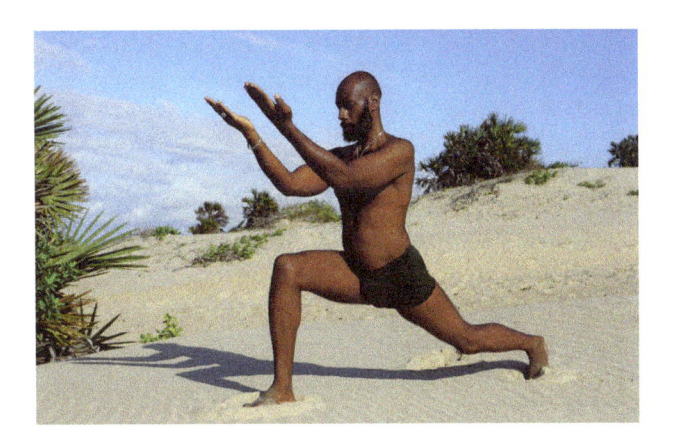

Physically

1. Promotes strength in legs
2. Develops flexibility in legs
3. Increases flexibility in the thighs, abdomen, and back
4. Increases flexibility in feet and toes
5. Increases strength in buttocks, feet, and ankles
6. Promotes and increases balance, posture in the back, legs, and spine
7. Opens the hips and groin area
8. Opens the chest and strengthens the shoulders
9. Increases mobility in the shoulder blades
10. Increases circulation in the organs and tones the abdominals

Mentally

1. Eliminates lethargy and laziness
2. Promotes strength of mind
3. Develops courage and fearlessness
4. Imparts resilience and strength

Ma'at

This Sanuy seems simple, yet it requires a high level of concentration and balance.

Stand with your feet shoulder-width apart; raise both arms from the sides laterally away from the body, keeping the fingers together stretching and pointing. Then turn the head to the right, followed by the feet, keeping the rest of the body facing forward to give a gentle twist in the spine. Bend the back foot going down on your knee, lean back, and sit on your back heel. Maintain the stretch in the arms, keeping them up, straight and leveled with your shoulders. Sit and breathe for three deep breaths.

Rise up and reverse each movement by turning the feet pointing forwards, then the head and lastly drop the arms down to the sides. Repeat the process by turning the head and the feet to the left.

The benefits of this Sanuy include:

Physically

1. Invigorates the circulation
2. Strengthens the shoulders
3. Increases flexibility in chest and shoulders
4. Stretches the thighs and knees
5. Increases stamina

Mentally

1. Develops determination, single-mindedness
2. Improves mental concentration and physical balance
3. Reduces mental stress
4. Alleviates anxiety

Ma'at helps the body to feel lighter and increases sekhemic flow to the lungs and heart.

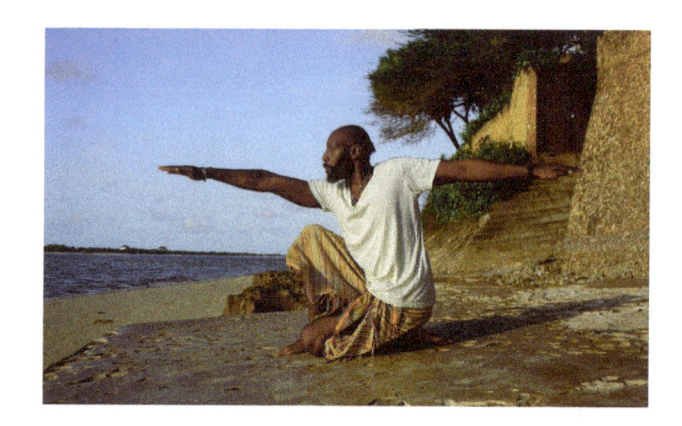

Aset

Stand with feet slightly apart and inhale. Raise both arms laterally and take a step back with the left leg. Bend the left knee going down on the knee, and lean back, sitting on the heel. Keep the back straight and the arms raised.

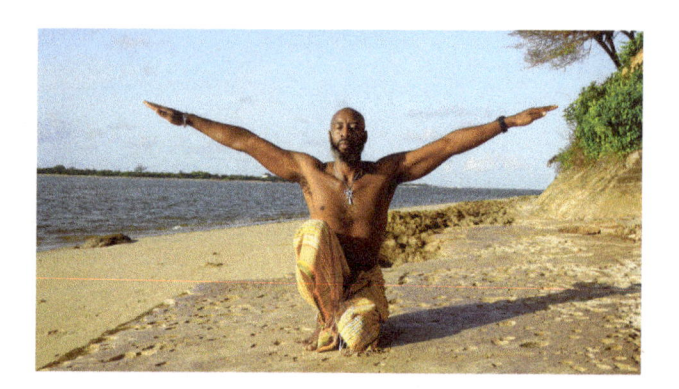

The benefits of this Sanuy include:

1. Strengthens shoulders and upper back
2. Strengthens thighs
3. Tones the abdominals
4. Opens the chest
5. Strengthens the ankles and toes
6. Develops balance

Contraindications

Ankle and knee injuries

Aset's Embrace

Stand legs shoulder-width apart and bring the arms out towards the sides, away from the body, stretching the chest and keeping the palms facing each other.

This can be a graceful movement with the use of the breath or it can be used as a form of dynamics or tension by tensing the arms, as you bring the palms to face each other in front of the torso. Once in this pose, contract the muscles of the back and release and relax the arms, moving lightly back to a wide arm stretch. Inhale as the arms are wide, and slowly exhale as the arms move forward and hands face downward and towards each other whilst tensing or resisting.

The benefits of this Sanuy include:

Physically

1. Improves circulation
2. Develops and stimulates the lungs
3. Strengthens the nervous system

Mentally

1. Promotes calm
2. Relieves stress and anxiety

Sekhemic

Strengthens the auric field

Increases eletro-magnetic energy

Increases Sekhem energy

Rejuvenates Sekhemic energy throughout the entire body

Djed Asaru

Begin by standing very straight, crossing the arms over your chest, right arm over left. Place the fingers on the collarbone. Close the eyes and concentrate on the spine. Gently push out the stomach and inhale for a count of four, and hold the breath for a count of two. Exhale slowly through the nose for a count of four, pulling the abdominals in. Rest for two counts. Keep the cycles of rhythmic breathing going in Djed Asaru with the arms crossed over the chest, as this position is a meditative state. The Sanuy creates a pyramid and is useful for the Heper (heart) and Ab (solar plexus) chakras, and for regenerative purposes. This pose can be used also to induce a deep, restful, and cell-stimulating sleep.

The benefits of this Sanuy include:

Physically

1. Rejuvenates the heart
2. Rejuvenates and stimulates the solar plexus

Mentally

1. Increases balance
2. Promotes concentration

Also, see Haru.

Establishment Sanuyaat

Rus Bagum Headstand

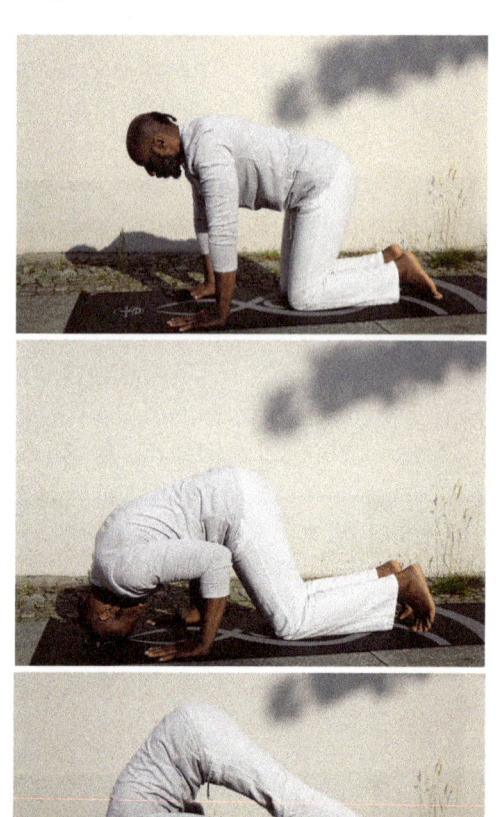

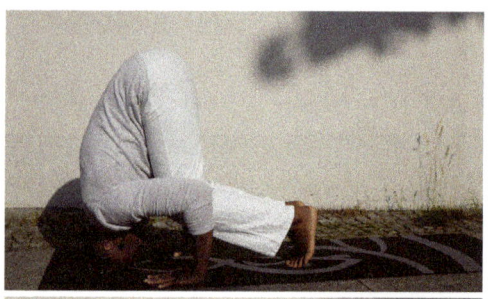

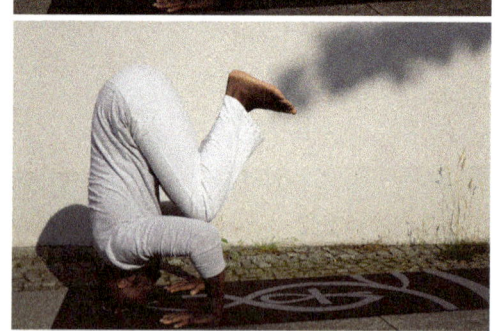

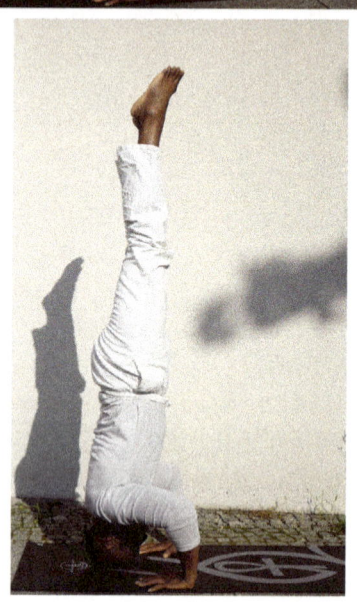

This advanced Sanuy is highly recommended for its development of concentration and the stimulation of the pineal gland – the melanin factory in your brain.

Begin with kneeling position Heru sitting. Place your arms on the mat and form an Aset Taruh/lock, widening your elbows so that you form a triangle shape with your forearms and hands, which are locked together via the fingers. Place your head inside the hands, rolling it so the back of your head is up against the inside of your fingers, and you are resting on the top of your head. Raise your body by stretching out your legs behind you and roll forward so you are now on top of your head. The alternative is to create a triangle with the hands and head, the head being at the top of the triangle.

Now inhale and walk your feet towards your elbows. Exhale and raise your feet off the ground, bending at the knee and pushing the feet straight upwards. Concentrate on perfection. Hold for 9-45 breaths. Inhale/exhale, come down, keeping your head on the ground and back to kneeling position. Then turn and lay on your back to let the blood naturally flow back to normal for a few moments.

The benefits of this Sanuy include:

Physically

1. Strengthens the respiratory system
2. Increases circulation
3. Rests the heart through gravity (returns the venous blood flow towards the heart)
4. Slows down the rate of the heartbeat and breathing
5. Rejuvenates the entire body

Mentally

1. Increases memory
2. Increases concentration
3. Stimulates intellectual capacity
4. Promotes the sensory capacities

Khepri/ Dub/scarab

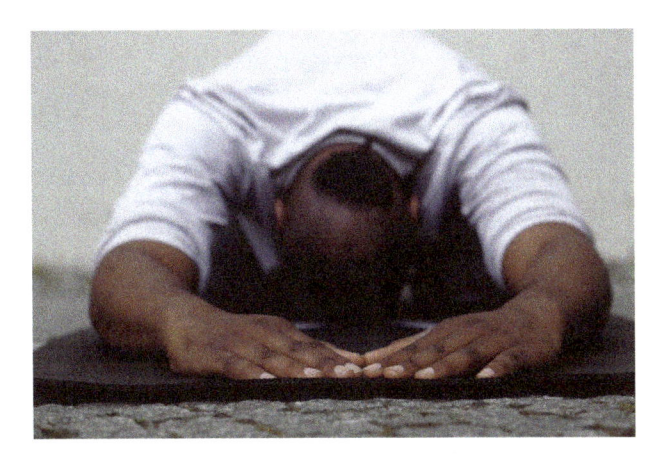

Sit on your heels with your shoulders nice and even. Bow forward and gently place your torso and upper body on your thighs, bring your arms forward and lengthen the arms, reaching forward. Stretch the sides of your body from your hips to your shoulders. Now allow the arms to go limp and relax, palms facing down.

As an option, you may draw the arms back towards your feet and let the shoulders widen, then turn the palms upward alongside your feet.

The benefits of this Sanuy include:

Physically

1. Alleviates the head, neck, and chest
2. Opens the pelvis, hips, and lower back
3. Stretches the ankles, knees, and hips
4. Opens up the upper back, relieving tension in the shoulders

Mentally

1. Calms the mind
2. Reduces stress and lessens fatigue

Contraindications

Do not do this if you have an ankle, knee or hip injury.

If pregnant, keep the knees apart and do not put too much pressure on your abdominals – a cushion or thick layer of blankets can be used between the abdominal region and thighs for support.

Asar/Karast (Mummy)

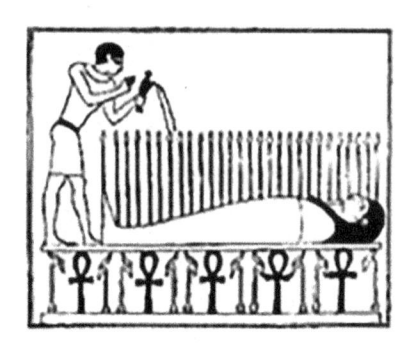

Lie flat on your back, eyes closed, legs slightly apart, with hands by your sides, palms facing upwards. Stay in this position for a minute or two. Concentrate on the breath. Take a long, slow inhalation, inviting the breath into your lungs and filling the upper body by applying mid and lower breathing. Hold the breath for a count of three; as you count, pull the Sekhem into every cell of your being. Exhale with complete control, nice and slow. Continue with this line of breathing up to nine breaths, expanding the rib cage and pushing the stomach up towards the ceiling. You can continue to breathe deeply but as normally as you can for a complete 10 mins. This Sanuy integrates the benefits of your yoga practice and allows the body to gather energy. The focus is on nurturing and centring yourself. You do this so that you may continue to nurture others in the world, sharing your peace, tranquility, and calm.

The benefits of the Sanuy include:

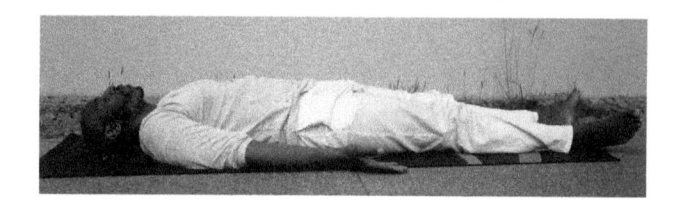

Physically

1. Increases lung capacity
2. Increases internal muscle control
3. Oxygenates the blood
4. Alkalizes the body
5. Detoxifies the body
6. Lowers blood pressure
7. Reduces fatigue
8. Triggers relaxation throughout the entire nervous system

Mentally

1. Calms the mind
2. Promotes tranquillity and ease
3. Produces a feeling of being nurtured
4. Rejuvenates the mind

Nefertum

The session is completed with meditation, sitting in Nefertum pose.

This can last between 10 mins to a full hour. (Please refer to meditation poses and meditation exercises from page 125.)

18 minutes Morning set

1. SHU

Stand erect and extend arms out, raise the arms overhead with thumbs touching, inhaling deeply as you raise arms and rise on to your toes.

Exhale YAA SHU slowly, as you drop arms and come back onto your feet. Repeat nine times slowly, increasing to 36 times (two minutes).

2. NUT

Raise arms overhead, thumbs touching and arch backwards, and exhale, slowly bend forward to touch toes. Repeat times slowly, increasing to 36 times (two minutes).

THESE TWO COMBINED CHARGE ELECTRO-MAGNETIC FIELD

3. WIDE LEG STRETCH

Sit and spread legs wide apart. Now forward bend to the centre for a few seconds.

Stretch towards the left foot and lower the head to the left knee, with deep Sekhem breath, hold for one minute.

Inhale, pull in the stomach and squeeze buttocks. Hold as long as possible and release, slowly exhaling.

Relax and repeat the stretch on the right side for one minute.

4. SELKET

On stomach, place forehead on the floor, mat or cushion, place hands palms down under thighs (beginners use fists).

And inhale, as you raise legs straight and high as possible and hold as long as possible. Exhale, lowering your legs.

Repeat for two minutes.
Relax for one minute.

5. WADJET/Arat

In supine position place hands palms down just under your shoulders.

Keep the elbows on the ground and close to your sides.

Turn the toes in and raise the chest off the floor, pushing upwards, using your hands, spread your fingers. Arching the torso up in cobra, concentrate on the third eye and turn your toes out. Inhale and exhale, holding as long as possible, keep the shoulders relaxed.

Repeat for as long as possible.
Continue for three minutes.
Relax for one minute.

6. GEB/The Plough

In supine position raise legs and hips perpendicular to the floor, supporting them with your hands and move into Katuf Bagum/Shoulder Stand, placing your weight onto your shoulders, neck and upper arms.

Keeping your legs straight, gently lower them down to the floor behind and away from the head. Hold for 30 seconds, increasing to one minute. Inhale and exhale.

Rest for one minute.

7. Easy Pose/Adept

Sit in the Easy pose and lie back with hands folded in Aset lock on the navel. Meditate on the third eye for two minutes. Increase according to your leisure.

This set raises the Sekhem energy and is an excellent preparation for meditation.

PATARUGSHIL-RE...
THE JOURNEY OF RE

Position 1.
Asaru/mummy

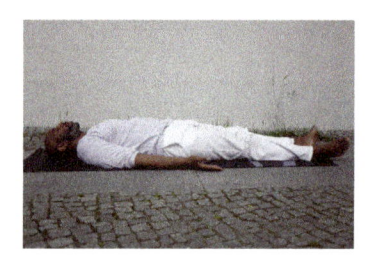

Position 2.
Taful Exhale

Prayer pose, the male and female energies coming together, balancing

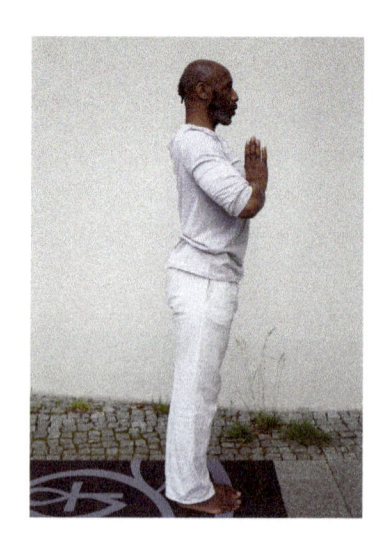

Position 3.
The Duat/Amenta Inhale

Backward bend

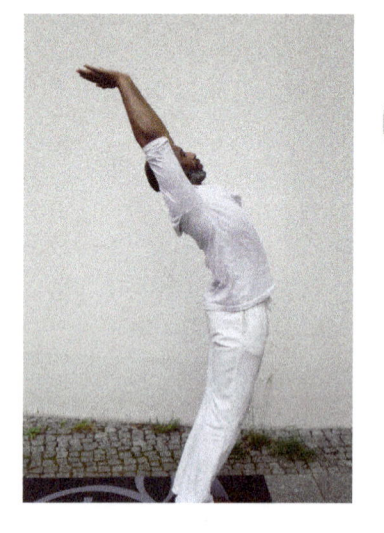

Position 4.
Standing Nut/Sky Exhale

Forward bend

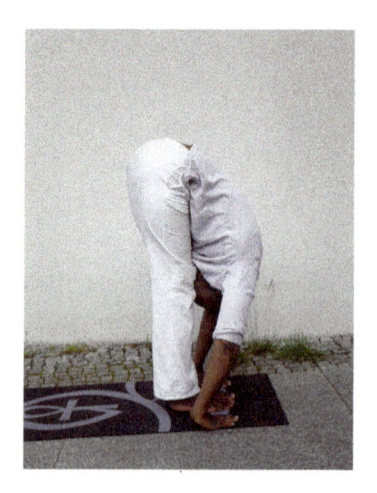

Position 5.
Right leg stretch Inhale

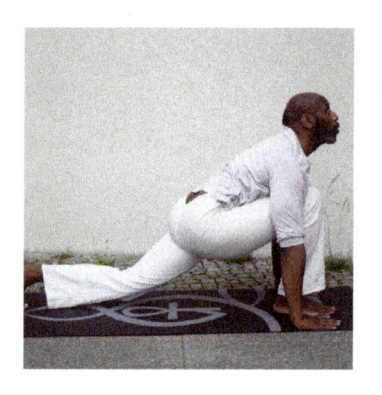

Position 6.
Pyramid Exhale

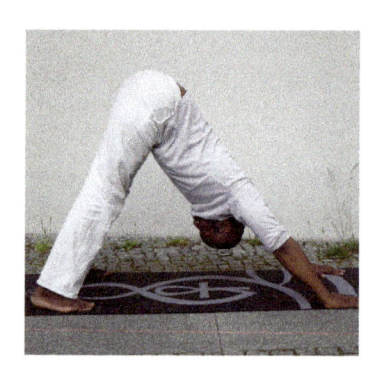

117 | THE RE-EMERGENCE OF TAMA-RE SMAI TAUI AFRIKAN YOGA

Position 7.
Arat/Cobra Inhale

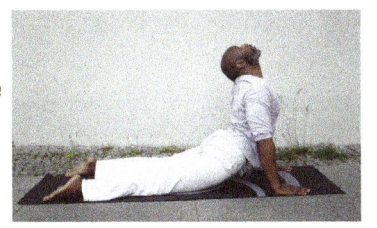

Position 8.
Heru Rising
Hold the breath

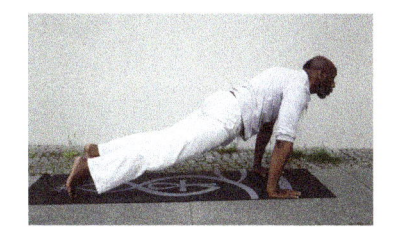

Position 9.
Pyramid Exhale

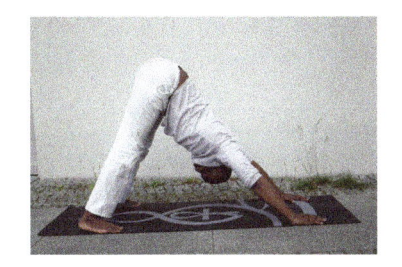

Position 10.
Leg stretch Inhale

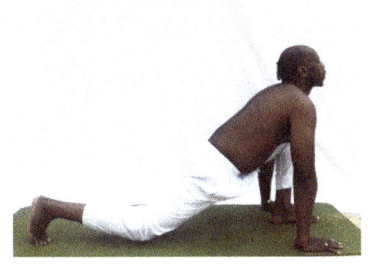

Position 11.
Nut Inhale into
Amenta Exhale

Repeat changing leg.

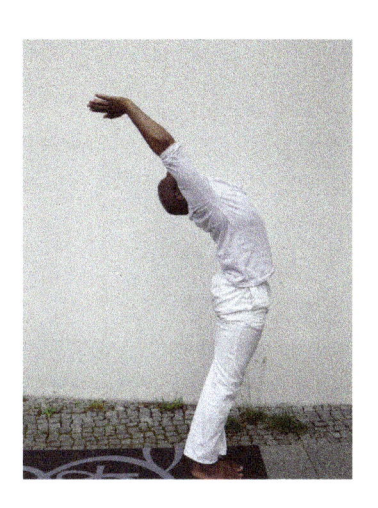

Patarugshil-Re...
The Journey of Re

Takes 3-10 minutes a day

All you need is a space measuring 2 square meters, and it costs nothing.

This acts on all the organism of the body and is not limited to one part only.

- **Patarugshil-re** tones up the digestive system by the alternate stretching and compression of the abdominal region. It massages the liver, the spleen, intestines, and kidneys, activating the digestion and getting rid of constipation and dyspepsia (disorders of the stomach).

- **Patarugshil-re** strengthens the abdominal muscles, the arms, and the wrists.

- **Patarugshil-re** synchronizes movement with breathing, thoroughly ventilating the lungs. It oxygenates the blood and acts as a de-toxicant because it gets rid of a large amount of carbon dioxide and other toxic gases through the respiratory tract.

- **Patarugshil-re** increases cardiac activity and the flow of blood throughout the system, which is ideal for the health of the body.

- **Patarugshil-re** combats hypertension and palpitations and warms up the extremities.

- **Patarugshil-re** tones up the nervous system by successfully stretching and bending the spine; it regulates the functions of the sympathetic and parasympathetic systems and helps to promote sleep.

- **Patarugshil-re** improves memory.

- **Patarugshil-re** relieves worry and anxiety.

- **Patarugshil-re** stimulates and normalizes the activity of the endocrine glands, the thyroid, in particular, through the movement of the neck.

- **Patarugshil-re** refreshes the skin, and, if done correctly, slight sweating and moisture may appear. Under African skies, a few minutes is enough. The skin will be well irrigated so that it reflects good health, and the complexion will clear.

- **Patarugshil-re** improves muscle structure throughout the body.

- **Patarugshil-re** strengthens neck, shoulders, arms, wrists, back, abdominals as well as the thighs, calves, and ankles without inducing hardening of the muscles.

- **Patarugshil-re** alleviates backache due to the strengthening of the back.

- **Patarugshil-re** in women and girls helps the bust develop normally. It becomes firm, regaining any loss in elasticity through stimulation of the glands and strengthening the pectoral muscles.

- **Patarugshil-re** controls activity in the uterus and ovaries, suppressing menstrual irregularity and accompanying pain; also assists in childbirth.

- **Patarugshil-re** increases immunity to diseases.

- **Patarugshil-re** provides grace and ease to the movements of the body, preparing the body for sports of all kinds.

- **Patarugshil-re** revives and maintains a spirit of youthfulness, producing health and strength, and longevity – an asset beyond price.

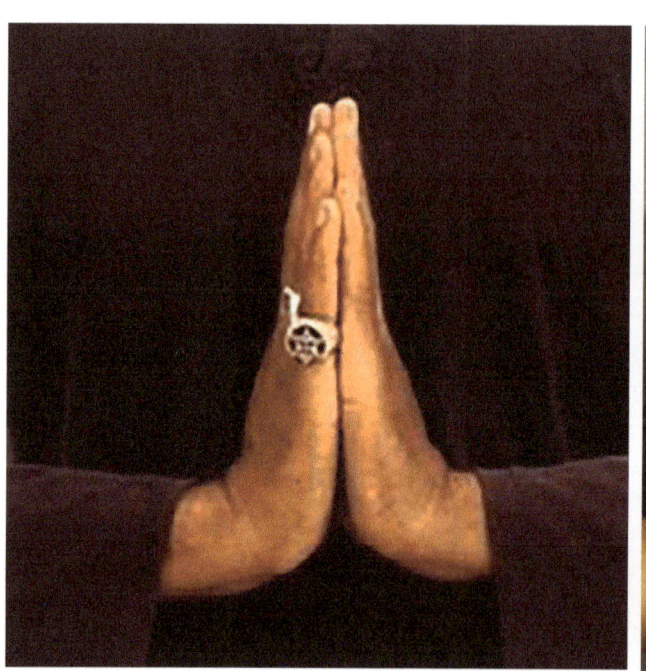

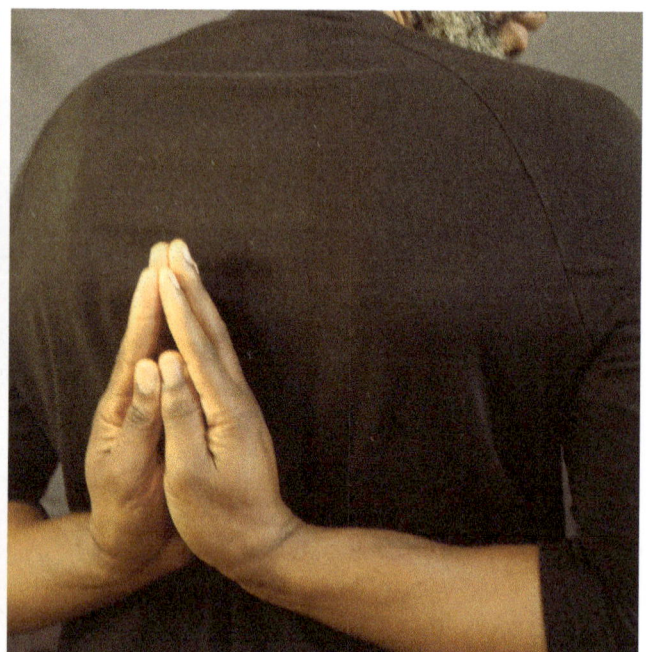

HAND **POSITIONS**

TARUH ISTAMZAAB

Hand gestures or position locks guide energy flow and reflexes to the brain. By curling, crossing, stretching and touching the fingertips to the thumb we can talk to the body and mind, as each finger corresponds with the different parts of the body and mind and is interlinked with psychic channels.

If you place enough pressure (but not so much that you whiten the fingertips), you will feel the flow of energy through these channels up the arms.

The thumb represents the ego.

Shu Taruh

Index finger: Jupiter
Stimulating knowledge
Ability
Organ: Lungs

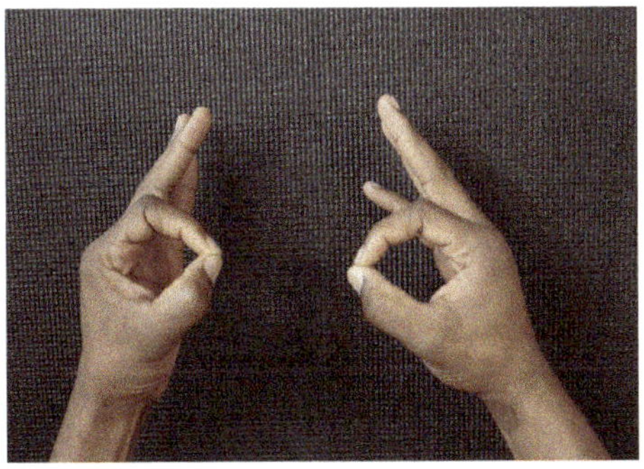

Aset Taruh

Middle finger: Saturn
Stimulating Patience
Nurturing
Organ: Liver

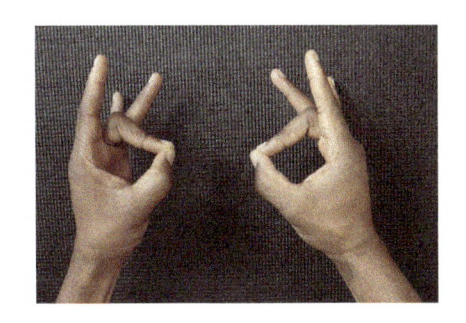

RE Taruh

Ring finger: Sun
Stimulating energy, health and intuition
Organ: Circulation/Sex

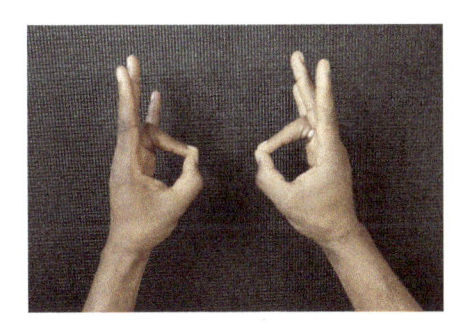

Anubu Taruh

Little finger: Mercury
Stimulating clear intuitive communication
Organ: Heart

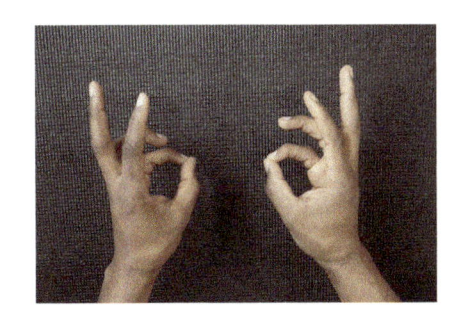

ASET LOCK/GRIP

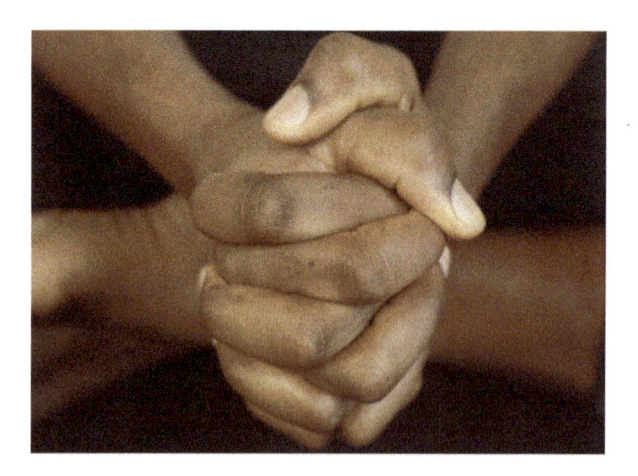

Taui / Taful Taruh

The Prayer / Union Pose – this is where both palms are pressed together, neutralizing and balancing both male and female principles for centering.

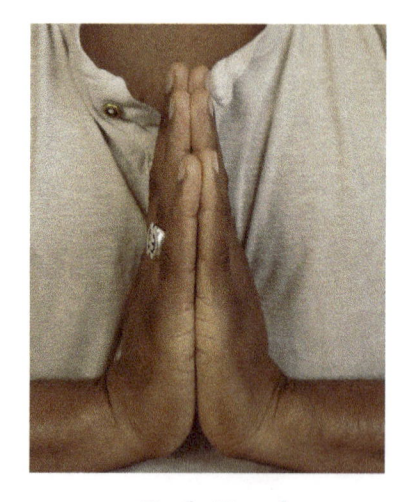

Ptah Taruh

The Prayer pose – this is where both palms are pressed together, neutralizing, and balancing both male and female principles for centering.

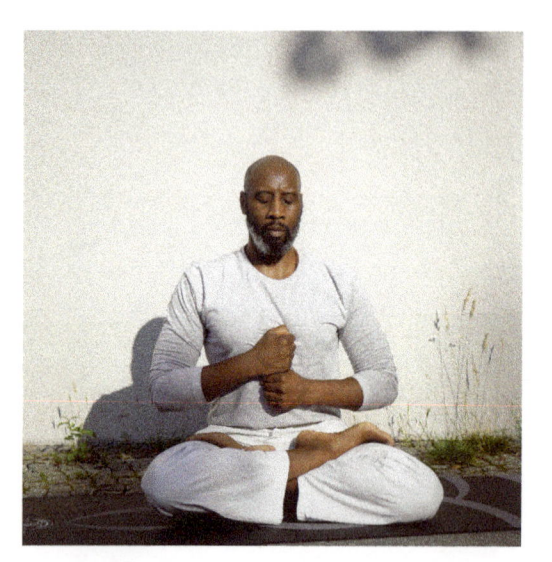

Both hands are curled into a fist, the left on the bottom and the right positioned on the top over and against the solar plexus/sternum, for stability, balance, and centering.

Finger	Planet	Zodiac	Supreme being/ Kosmic energy	Body
Index	Jupiter	Sagittarius	Shu	Lungs/thighs
Middle	Saturn	Capricorn	Aset	Liver/bones/knees
Ring	Sun	Leo	Re/Het-Heru	Circulation/sex
Little	Mercury	Virgo/Gemini	Anubu	Heart

Chant & Hand gestures

Sound AH MUN RE TA

Ah : touch index finger to the thumb (index = Shu, stimulating knowledge and ability).

Mun : touch the middle finger to the thumb (middle = Aset, patience and giving patience).

Re : touch the ring finger to the thumb (ring = RE/Hathor, giving energy, health, and intuition).

Ta : little finger to the thumb (little = Anubu, clear and intuitive communication).

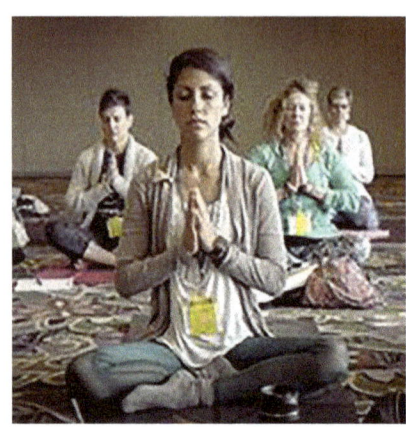

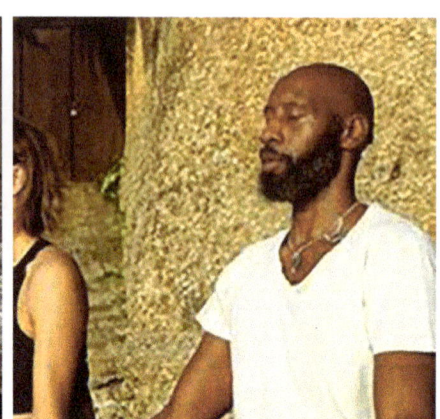

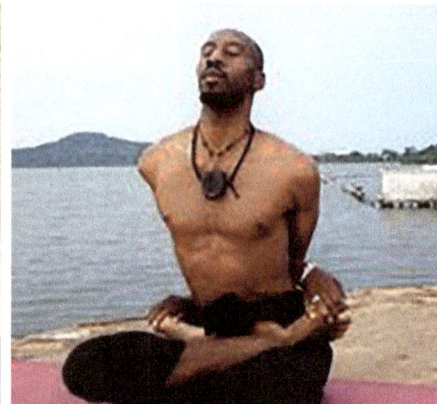

MEDITATION

"Live in truth. Enter silence. There is peace. Peace is silence."

The Mind, Scroll 11:53 inscribed by Dr Malachi Z York

125 | THE RE-EMERGENCE OF TAMA-RE SMAI TAUI AFRIKAN YOGA

The Afrikan Yoga, Hudu, and Hanuaat/exercises are meditation through movement; and this form of meditation is very useful for the active, rapid mind.

However, meditation through stillness is useful for those who wish to search deeper into the constructs of the soul. This search is to find self and tap into the source of all things, thereby generating internal healing and mental manifestations of the will on a cosmic, etheric and holistic level.

The Smai student/practitioner must be one or he/she will be many, and with many comes confusion, not just for him/her, but whomever he/she comes in contact with, creating turmoil and chaos. We are unaware of this, so we go about wreaking havoc in people's lives, thinking we are doing good deeds. This is the mistake of many good-doers, leaders, ministers, priests, teachers, and those who claim to be healers. We must be one, centred, and balanced or we will walk around with the many in our heads, bringing confusion.

Meditation is simply an observation of the mind. The practitioner is being a witness of self now centering and controlling the mind. (Please refer to The 9 Principles of Tehuti Mental on page 38.) Meditation is mind control via the self through internal means rather than the numerous forms of mind control via external means. There is much to be said about meditation with much of it focused on theory, so here are a few exercises to actually experience meditation.

The key thing is to be completely relaxed. Sit in a comfortable position so you can be still for a period of 10 minutes to one hour.

Breath Meditation

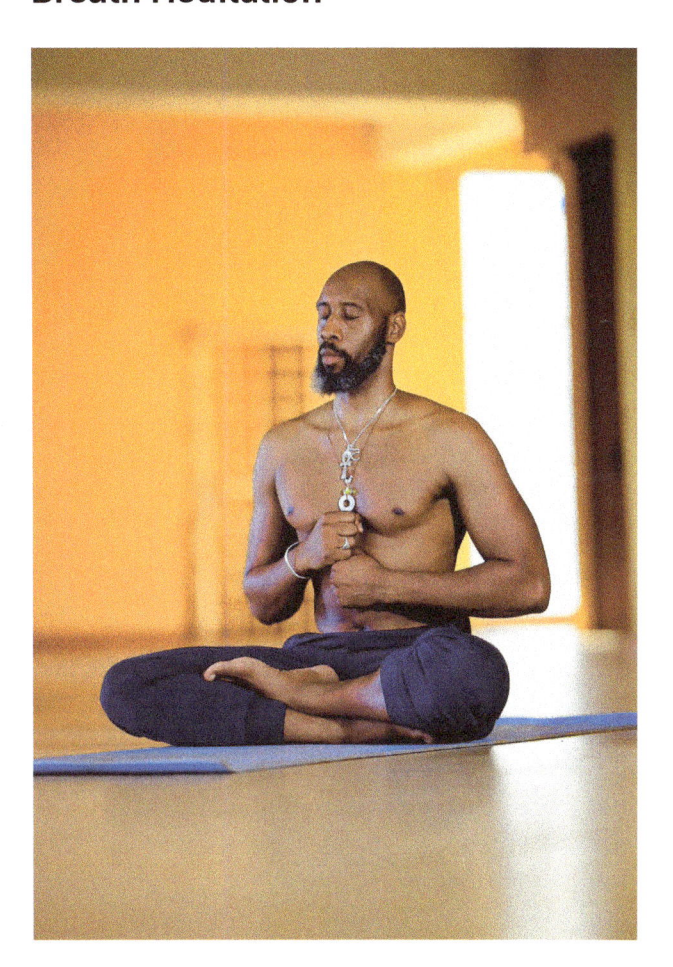

Sit on a chair or on the floor if you can cross the legs. (Please refer to Sitting Sanuyaat for Meditation on page 96.) Pull your spine upwards and make the spine tall. Close the eyes and concentrate on the flow of air entering the nostrils. Visualize the flow rolling down into the abdomen, filling the torso and pushing the abdomen out. Feel the air brush all around your nose and feel it flow out on the exhale. Allowing the abdomen to deflate, gently pull the abdomen back towards the spine. This movement of breath is the first stage as it slows down and begins to focus the mind on the 'Arush Shiru', nasal chakra. This also stimulates the Mer seat in between the eyebrows, opening the first eye, the Eye of Horus.

The other Arushaat will begin to open – do not be concerned – for this meditation is simply to observe the breath and by doing so to narrow down the many ramblings of the mind into one gleaming instrument. Oneness is the attainment.

The mind will drift, and you will be bombarded with many thoughts. Do not worry, just gently guide the mind back to the breath and inhale, and exhale the air through the nostrils. With practice, the concentration will develop. Give yourself time and nurture yourself.

Now Meditation

The mind has a tendency to live in the future or the past; in fact, most of us are in that state most of the time and therefore unconscious. Unconscious because the past is not real, it has gone, and you cannot get it back. In the now it does not exist. The future has not happened yet, and many of us worry about and project to events we feel may be of concern, or wonderful happenings that do not really exist in the now. 'The Now' is real. Meditation assists your conscious awareness of this fact.

Sit on a chair or on the floor. Keep the spine and head erect just as in the Breath meditation. Close the eyes and concentrate on the flow of breath entering the nostrils. Breath steadily and observe your mind – it will begin to wonder either to the past or the future. By observing the mind's journey, you will be aware of the illusory state. Ask yourself this, "Where am I right now?" This can also be useful when doing a task and the mind wonders therefore cutting your energy and concentration down to a small percentage, the question becomes, "What am I doing right now?" The mind will automatically answer, and you will be gently brought back to a state of now. You may have to do this a few times in a session. The Smai student uses this process to be present in any situation.

Candle Meditation

This form of meditation is for concentration, visualization and exercising the first eye (The Mer Arush). It is also useful for children to develop stillness and focus. Alternatively, you can use a small object or a dot on the wall.

Sit, using the seated poses for meditation, a few feet away from a candle and focus on the flame. The breath must remain steady and rhythmic. Watch the flame dance and flicker – all of your periphery vision will begin to narrow down as you enter into the flame. Slowly narrow the eyes until they naturally close. Keep the image of the flame in the forefront of your mind. This forefront will be between your eyebrows – the seat of the first eye, 'The eye of Heru' (The Mer Arush). Keep this focus for as long as you can and use the breath to go into yourself; using the first eye to look within, you will find a place of no-mind, stillness, and peace.

SUGGESTIONS
FOR A BENEFICIAL PRACTICE

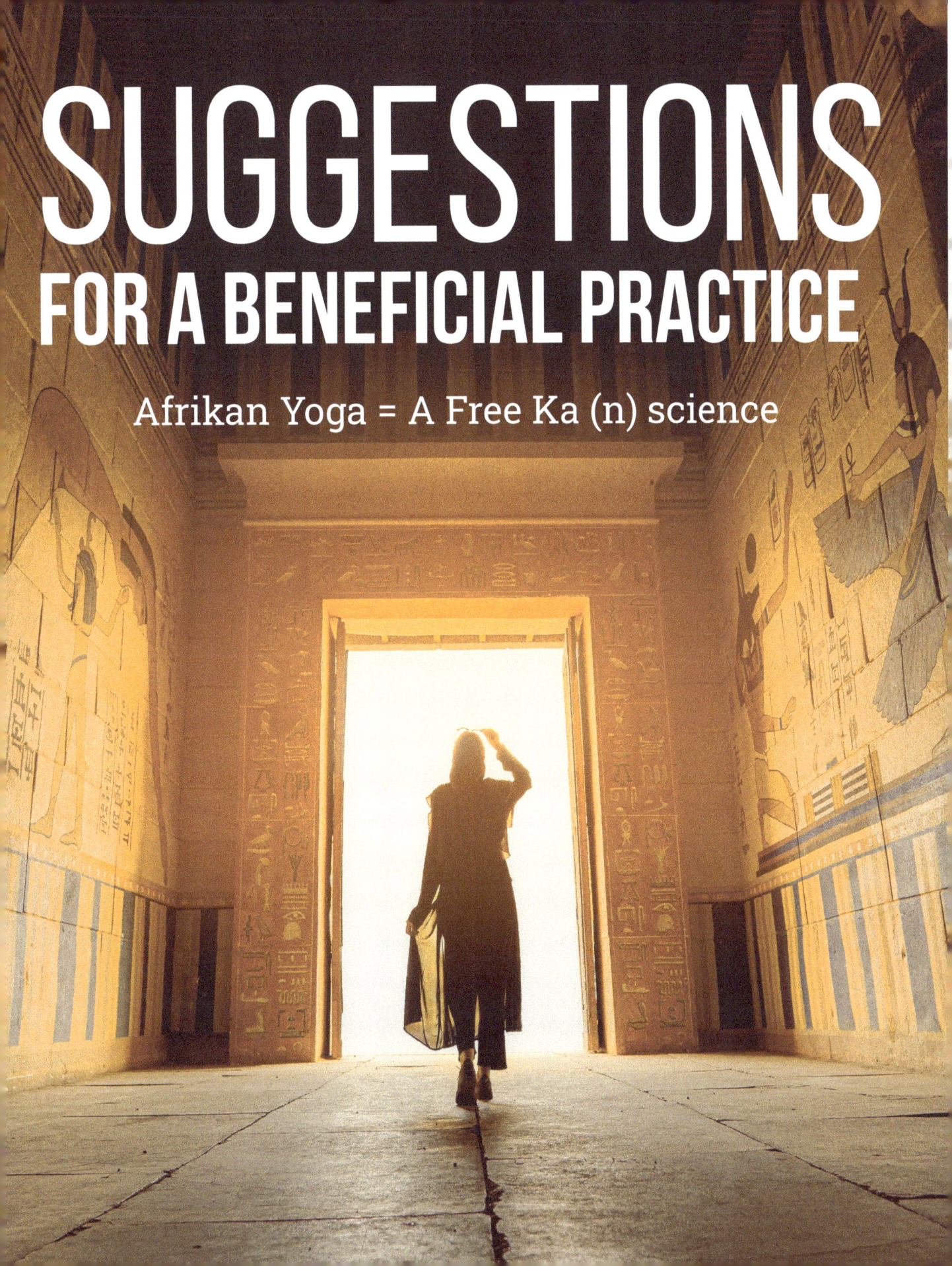

Afrikan Yoga = A Free Ka (n) science

An affirmation:

To my mental and physical efforts, I add the potential of my spiritual self. Its qualities permeate affairs. Its powers flow through my entire being.

Time and Patience

Time is relevant to one's state of consciousness. What do I mean by that? When one is young and full of energy with apparently very little to do, and the concentration span is low, time appears to be long. On the other hand, when one is older and has mastered the art of concentration through meditation, the energy is retained to achieve much, time appears quicker. Another example, you are in an aerobics class jumping up and down to some pumping music. Your heart is thumping and your lungs have ballooned to the point where they feel they are going to pop. It's an hour-long class, and you have only done 10 minutes. The next day you attend a yoga class and are asked to stretch, concentrating on your breath, your muscles, and blood. You are asked to nurture yourself and take it easy. All the movements are slow and deliberate, yet the class finishes before you are even aware – and this is an hour and a half class. What appears to be long is actually short because one's state of consciousness has shifted.

So time is down to consciousness: the higher the consciousness, the shorter the time to the point where time and space cease to exist. This point is known as God-consciousness or tapping into the seventh plane of existence. So there are many time zones that are not based on geographic location but on varied states of existence and consciousness. Take time in your practice and you'll find that you move from zone to zone, state to state, and that your mentality can accommodate much more as it expands. At the same time, time is sped up to the point (the black dot) that time and space cease to exist. You are one with 'All', here and there at the same time. Einstein and other scientists understood that the key to time travel was to move at the speed of light. This is what you do when your consciousness shifts – you become more of a light being, less solid. Why? Because your cells have sped up. This works with the breath, meditation and Sanuyaat. The best time for a beneficial practice is in the morning before 8 am assisting the awakening of the body and mentally preparing and stimulating the practitioner for the rest of the day. You can also practise during the evening, before going to bed. However, make this light and shorter as the stretches you use should in no way be overdone because the muscles and the body want to rest, and therefore exertion can cause injury.

It is also advised not to rush your forms or to compete with others at achieving the desired outcomes of postures. Take time and use time, be patient and secure in the knowledge you have gained to date. Use this book to understand what is happening to the body and mind, use the Neteru to gain benefits of nature and always be good to yourself.

Nutrition

The golden rule is not to be excessive or overindulgent in certain foods and drinks, like spicy foods, sugary and salty foods, alcohol, and drinks that dehydrate the body. The benefit of adequate nutrition is the general homeostasis of the body, providing health and vitality. The consumption of high amounts of sugar can prove to be lethal. A spoon of white refined sugar can lower the immune system by 70 per cent. Now, none of the bodily systems and organs functions separately or independently of each other. So how can we assume that the function of the brain and the psychological, and emotional processes will not be adversely affected by a substance that is able to affect the performance of the liver, pancreas, lungs, kidneys, gall bladder, spleen, or heart, and other organs? Think of it this way: sugar erodes the teeth, one of the hardest substances in the body. Smai practitioners have found that food affects the subconscious mind and one's physical and mental performance.

Sugar, in particular, dulls the positive capacity of the spirit in ways you could only imagine. An example of this is eating a sugary snack before going to bed can result in a dream, where you are on the run from someone or something, fighting someone or something or witnessing violent actions. These are ripples in the brain circuitry caused by the overwork of the pancreas and adrenals processing the sugar in your digestive system. When overstressed, these organs and glands are likely to sympathetically produce adrenaline – the commonly known chemical substance associated with 'fight or flight'. Sugar stimulates the secretion of adrenaline, and you are in a battle during the time of rest.

You are in a state of fear, and this can happen any time during the day or night. The divine energy and grace that we travel with are nullified through the intake of particular substances that are termed as 'pica'/non-food. Today in modernity – another way of saying western – we are saturated with man-made substances labelled as 'food'.

The Smai practitioner learns to curb the urges of working against nature in this manner or suffers the consequences immediately. The Smai practitioner understands that fresh vegetables and fruit or the lack of them go an extremely long way in effectively making an impact on their health and the health of their community. No matter what social class or ethnicity, fresh food cannot be undervalued as a key factor in the health of individuals. Fruit and vegetables carry high amounts of nutrients, vitamins and water in a formula that the body can easily absorb to sustain and maintain homeostasis and cellular function. Fruit and vegetables grown by 'Re' sunlight in organic soil are the best sources of bodybuilding on the planet. This source is not just for the body, organs, and cellular functions; it also has an effect on how you think, process information, and form human relationships. Amunnubi Ruakh Ptah taught that, *"Improper diet is another hindrance to spiritual progress. All foods have distinct energies, just as the physical body is formed from the gross physical portions of the foods that are eaten. So the mind is formed from the subtler portions. If the food is impure, the mind also becomes impure."*

He goes on to say, **"What goes into the human body correlates directly to the efficiency with which the brain functions. Recent studies show, that certain red food colourings create hyperactivity in children and that refined sugar can cause emotional instability, and this is what most parents are starting their children on."**

In a *Guardian* article dated 03/11/04:

A study led by the Harvard school of public health in Boston analysed data from more than 100,000 health professionals over 14 years and concluded such a diet [a diet of fruit and vegetables] led to a 'modest' overall reduction in chronic disease, largely because of the impact on preventing heart disease and strokes.

The Department of Health has said increasing fruit and vegetable consumption is the most important anti-cancer measure after stopping people smoking.

Green leafy vegetables were strongly associated in a US research study with lowering the risk of cardiovascular disease. Those participants that ate at least 5 servings of fruits and vegetables daily had a lower risk (28 per cent) of vascular disease than participants eating fewer than 1.5 portions a day, probably due to the higher intake of nutrients which were not destroyed through cooking. I have found from personal experience, that when I take fresh fruit and green leafy vegetables eaten raw, I am vibrant, have more energy, am mentally sharper, and far more sensitive to my surroundings. I have seen similar potency in others with the same eating habits.

Drink Water

Water is ultimately a purifying detoxifying chemical. We are in fact more water beings than earthlings. Our bodies are 70 to 75 per cent water – some say more than that, and each part of our body right down to the cellular level needs water.

Drinking plenty of water flushes out toxins and baths internal organs. The oxygen regenerates and assists the body's absorption of food, improving the digestive system and other systems of the body.

Water carries electricity; electro-neuron impulses are the fundamental premise of the nervous system. The entire human nervous system consists of these electro-neuron impulses carrying messages to and from the brain. It functions well with the correct amount of plain water. Drink 6-8 glasses per day to maintain the body's natural equilibrium.

Deep Breathing

A human can do without food for well over a week and up to a month. A human can do without water for days, yet a human is unable to function without air for only a few minutes. This is the magnanimous importance of breath.

The majority of western society practises improper breathing which causes respiratory problems and diseases of the body. Breathing from the chest (Tat shallow breathing) and insufficient use of the diaphragm are the main components of western breathing practices. The Smai yogi uses **Deep Breathing,** using their whole diaphragm.

Deep Breathing improves bronchial function, providing good healthy lung tissue through the proper use of all portions of the lungs, preventing colds. It also improves the quality of the blood. The proper oxygenation of the blood is vital for adequate body function and a strong immune system. Every part of the body is dependent upon blood for nourishment. Proper breathing gently massages the internal organs, stimulating their actions, encouraging normal function. The diaphragm is nature's principal instrument for this internal exercise. Deep breathing gives you greater control of your body, increasing circulation, developing your mental capabilities, promoting the spiritual side of your nature. Lastly, deep breathing simply reduces stress.

Rest and Relaxation

Rest is an important aspect of life, as in the principle of rhythm one cannot be on the go all the time, and you will have to stop. For many in the city, this stopping tends to be against one's own will in the form of sickness and disease.

To avoid this, we must return to the laws of nature (Neteru), meaning to apply relaxation as a part of our way of life. This means relaxing physically and mentally and not just in front of the television. Relaxation is described as the absence of tension or the absence of muscular contraction. Tension is tightness or a stressed state. Tension is mental thoughts translated into action.

When relaxing, the Smai student should not imagine a strenuous activity like climbing a mountain or similar as thoughts are translated into physical action. He or she will utilize mountaineering muscles by generating the increased contraction of those particular muscles through thought, thereby defeating the aim of relaxation. It is easier to relax during exhalation than during inhalation as exhalation takes place during the relaxation of the large diaphragm muscle. When the diaphragm muscle is relaxed, the whole body tends to relax and let go of its tension. This exhalation is a release of all tension generally. As we exhale, we should relax more each time. Relaxation then becomes more progressive and deepened. Imagination plays a very large part in relaxation. By shaping images and making suggestions to the subconscious mind, it absorbs these subtle intentions of relaxation and implements them. By creating sensory images of the body becoming relaxed, the body will automatically become relaxed. When relaxing, the sensation of lightness and weightlessness follows the sensation of extreme heaviness. There are those who can only relax after a stretch – that is to say that stretching actually permits the muscles to relax and weeds out any further tension.

Sleep

According to nature's (Neteru) laws, we need a certain amount of relaxation. Unfortunately, for many of us, this only comes in the form of sleep. Sleep is a wonderful mechanism of nature, which western man still tries to defy for the sake of pleasure and recreation. The masters of relaxation tend to be children. Children have so much vigour, life and energy – when it is time to relax or sleep, see how fast they can lock of all activities and allow themselves to go into such a deep sleep they can be carried over rough terrain and not wake up until they are satisfied. See how utterly limp they become and how they sink into the couch, chair or bed, leaving an imprint – it is best to take a leaf out of their book in the art of relaxation. The thorough rest allows them to be completely within themselves and gives them the power to be so full of energy.

There are adults who also have the ability to relax completely. They tend to be calm and serene, not allowing agitating thoughts to take them into deepened states of worry and anxiety. The most successful business people have this tendency as they take the time to rest from work or have a power nap (snooze) during working hours, rejuvenating themselves to work in a jovial non-irritated manner.

Sleep for an adult is around 8 hours (Horus), and for a child, it is close to 12 hours.

This is so the body can rejuvenate, and cells replenish without the destruction we put it through whilst awake or in action.

This period of sleep is recommended to be one of the most nourishing on earth, and even more so if it is done in complete darkness between 10 pm and 6 am. The darkened state is important as any form of external light, such as light from a street lamp or bathroom, or hall lamp, even the little red light that's often beaming from some electric item in your bedroom, can affect the rich flow of melatonin from the pineal gland.

The Smai student does not really sleep – the Smai practitioner rests and regenerates. A technique used to maintain youth and vigour in the city through sleep is to take a black sheet and cover your bedroom window. All electricity must be switched off, and the room must be pitched in complete darkness.

To go further, one may sleep on his/her back, arms crossed over his/her chest, right over left, in the form of Asar (Osiris), thereby creating a pyramid. Science has already proven that organic objects placed within a pyramid structure decay far slower.

Positive Affirmations

Affirmation = A FIRM(ing) ATION (action-doing).

Making one resilient in self-belief and self-knowing.

Affirmation is the stabilising transference of self in a context through word sound.

"As a man thinks in his heart so is he" (or so he becomes).

Our belief systems do determine to an extent how our lives are run.

A positive attitude will produce positive results in our lives.

Our thoughts are the catalyst of our creations on a physical level.

They form our abundance or our lack, our achievements and our failures. Thoughts have weight, shape, form and colour.

That is why a positive affirmation thought (intent) and word sound are so relevant to balanced health. Unknowingly, we say affirmations every day when we put ourselves down. Phrases such as, "I don't think I can do that", "I'm not good enough", and "I'm ugly" will inform what you become. Our very cells and genes can be transformed with it. It is a very powerful instrument.

Positive uses of Affirmations

An affirmation is used to help you achieve your goals, and the key element is to place yourself in the now when you use your affirmation.

"I must become a better businessman" or "I will become a better businessman" still keeps you outside the door not crossing the threshold of change and transformation.

"I am a better businessman" takes one immediately across the threshold.

The intent of the affirmation is a crucial element; any space for doubt will throw the effect of a positive affirmation off, confusing the mind and body. Affirmations are said after a meditation or Smai session/practice when one has been centralized by these particular activities. The key is to be in a balanced state so that the conscious and unconscious minds work together in harmony. Remember, whatever you send out to mother-father universe in thought, the Kosmos universe sends back to you.

Principles, Causes, Movement/Vibration

"Our ultimate goal is to liberate our spirit from the compulsion of all conditions superimposed upon it" – Ra Nefer Amen

	Body/Disease	**Emotion**	**Hika/Posture**
Love	Cancer, Eczema, Eyes, Rheumatism, Left side of the body	Victimized, Chronic Bitterness, Resentment, Self-punishment, Rejection of feminine energy and processes	**Hika** Yaa Sobek Yaa Het-Heru Yaa **Aset** *"I lovingly release the past, they are free, and I am free."* **Posture** Ma'at, Aset, Wings of Aset
Freedom/Courage	Thyroid, Hips, Back, Body odour, Skin, Frigidity, Joints, Knees, Sciatica, Pre-menstrual syndrome, Cholesterol, Oedema	Humiliation, Fear related to money or the future, Being hypocritical	**Hika** Yaa Sakhmet *"I move into my greater good. My good is everywhere. I am secure and safe."* *"I bend and flow with life."* **Posture** Katuf Bagum/ Shoulder Stand Geb the Plough Shen the Wheel

Action	Hips, Constipation, Glands	Procrastination, Fear of moving forward	**Hika** Yaa Sakhmet **Posture** Manjet, Sitting Nut, Selket, Henu Ra Herukhuti
Wisdom	Pituitary, Bones, Bladder, Cancer, Dizziness, Feet, Left side of the body	Control, Anxiety, Rejection of feminine energy and processes, Lack of receptivity, Confusion	**Hika** Yaa Khonsu Yaa Haru **Posture** Nefertum Djed Asaru
Knowledge	Pituitary, Brain tumour, Prostate, Right side of the body	Control, Mental fears, Weakened masculinity, Belief in aging	**Hika** Yaa Shu "I balance my masculine energy easily & effortlessly." **Posture** Ma'at, Djed Asaru Headstand
Transcendence	Bedwetting, Sciatica, Right side of the body	Fear of the future, Issues with father, brother or male person	**Hika** Yaa Khonsu Yaa Haru **Posture** Djed Asaru
Power	Solar plexus, Anxiety, Cancer, Cellulite, Knees, Feminine fat problems, Obesity, Impotency, Venereal disease, Pre-menstrual syndrome, Spinal problems, Right side of the body	Stored anger, Self-punishment, Guilt, Lack of support, Pride, Ego	**Hika** Yaa Kek **Posture** Geb Spinal Twist Sons of Heru/Geb 4 points, Wadjet Cobra

Truth	Bowels, Circulation, Ears—Deafness, Knees, Eczema	Fear, Stubbornness, Inflexibility	**Posture** Sitting Nut Ma'at
Joy	Blood—Anaemia, Epilepsy, Cancer, Diabetes, Heart, Hips, Wrists, Eyes, Throat, Eczema	Fear of life, Feelings of 'not good enough', Lives in an unpleasant past	**Hika** Yaa Bes "I am balance, and free. I move forward in life with ease and joy." **Posture** Fire movement, Sebek, Het Heru

Epilogue

Remember, mastery is not about being picture perfect and therefore incapable of surrendering oneself to the desires of mortals. That means as a master, you still can find yourself in powerless situations, sulk, get angry or even scoff at others. Mastery is not the inability to fall or trip. Mastery is being able to transform and transcend the challenges of irritation, frustration, self-righteousness, and doubt, as the inevitable will appear. Mastery is acknowledging your capabilities and working those abilities to their full capacity to reach the next level.

Once mastery is achieved, there is a point of being. Just being. And this being can come at any point in your life beyond your life situation. Primarily, it must be understood that you have the power right now to achieve this point. 'Now' being the operative word—not when you go to a class or wait for the next teacher to come along: it must be understood that you and your life situations are that teacher. You and your life situations are the initiation and the journey to being. On this journey you, no doubt, will come across pain, suffering, internal turmoil and confusion due to the lack of self-awareness, ego and the laws of vibration, polarity, gender, etc. Yet this is also a marvellous time as it gives you the opportunity to let go. See the hopelessness and emptiness of the life filled with ego, desire and hankering. Once you want to change this in your life, then and only then are you ready for Smai/Yoga as you are ready to die and be reborn by experiencing the flip side to the negativity. The master chooses to experience joy, abundance, love, peace, beauty, oneness and clarity because this is the true reality of life, utilizing the very same divine principles.

There are ones who have arrived at the titles 'master', 'teacher' or 'leader' and even people in general who seek to manipulate other human beings and environments, etc., by way of knowledge, energy and vibration. Those who manipulate are also susceptible to manipulation for it is a sphere that has to be entered, and therefore all are subject to the laws of manipulation. The master alchemist exits the sphere of external relationships and enters the sphere of internal self. The master manipulates the subtle elements within him/herself and his/her external environment, thus human relationships are transformed. This is the way of the master who seeks self-mastery (internal self). Gautama Buddha says, "The master's function is to help you remember who you are."

"Hotep ila antuk, Hotep ila kull, peace to you, peace to all."

NOTES

For more information and involvement with PIMAY Afrikan Yoga School, Retreats and healthy living programmes, visit: www.pabloimanimethod.com

For bookings, workshops and presentations contact
Pablo M Imani: info@pabloimanimethod.com

GLOSSARY AND DEFINITIONS

A

Afrika	A free Ka (spirit) descendent of 9 ether / solar beings
Africa	'To divide'
African	Divided person
A'afrekan	African
Afrekeya	Africa
Amun	Hidden One / Neter
Amenta	Duat, the abode of Neter and the soul / the unconscious
Ankh	Key to life / key of the eternal
Anu	I Am / The Heavenly One
Anubu	Messenger of Heaven and Hell
Arush	Chakra
Arushaat	Chakras
Arat	Cobra
Asaru	'He who is seen' / The Eye
Aset	Throne, seat; also known as Isis
Atum	The undifferentiated one / first born of the deities
Atun	The unique one
Aum	(Nuwaupic) Sound of Life

B

Ba	'Strength, powerful' / soul
Bast	Cat / fire
Bayna	Mid breathing
Bes	Repeller of wrong doers

D

Djed	Stability
Djehuty	Tehuti / Thoth
Dub	Scarab beetle

E

Ennead	The Sacred Nine Neteru
Ethiopian	9 ether being, Kushite
Ether	Upper air, the medium of light and electromagnetism

F

Fug	High breathing

G

Gaanum	Chanting

H

Hanu	Movement
Hatha	Sun and moon / Het-Heru
Hekau/Hikau	Words of power
Heru	'Far away' hero / Horus
Hery Heb	Egyptian teachers
Het-Heru	The dwelling house of Horus
Hudu	Afrikan Tai Chi
Hika	One of the constant companions of Re; personification of miracles, magic and the manipulation of elements and chemicals
Huhi	The eternal breath
Hu	The force of creative will
Huwa	The creative force of will
Hotep	Peaceful, tranquil, satisfied

I

Isis	'Emotions'
Istamzaab	Position
Ifa	Yoruba Oracle system, the cosmic intelligence of Yoruba cultural expression
Indus Kush	Ancient name of India

K

Ka	'Double' spirit
Karast	Christ / anoint
Khat	Body
Khaybet	Plasmatic you
Kemet	The black one
Khemet	Land of the Blacks
Khemetic	Black culture
Khonsu	Traveler / healer
Khu	'Flail' mental

Kush	'Black' son of Ham, the father of Nimrod
	The name for Ethiopia before it was Abyssinia

M

Ma'at	Justice, order, righteousness / female personification of wisdom
Manjet	The morning boat of Ra/Re
Mutalub	Student

N

Nefertem	Lotus 'beautiful completion' Young Temu
NTR	Neter male/female
Neter	Male personification of a deity
Netert	Female personification of a deity
Neteru	Guardians / nature
Neb	Master
Nebu	Master
Nuwaubu	Right knowledge, right wisdom, right overstanding, sound right seasoning. 'News bringer'
Nuwaubian	A person who prescribes to 'right knowledge, right wisdom, right overstanding, sound right reasoning. A bringer of news'
Nubia	Land of the Nubians/Sudan
Nubun	Before the light, presenter of the news
Nun	The deep abyss
Nut	'Nurturer' Sky Netert

O

Osiris	'Lord of the perfect Black'
Orisha	(Yoruba) Neterian emanations of the creator manifesting through nature
Overstand	Oppose to understand—to stand above a situation, to get the 360 degrees of information and transcend

P

Pa	The Definitive
Ptah	Opener: 'one who opens the way'

R

Ra	Sun solar energy / life force: 'The creative power to make'
	Ragul Exercise

Ragulaat	Exercises
Re	'Sun's rays', Ra, Father, Sun deity

S

Sanuy	Form / posture
Sanuyaat	Forms / postures
Sebek	'He who reunites', to make pregnant
Sekhmet	The powerful, the mighty
Sem	Title of a priest 'Listener', 'A Hearer'
Shen	To encircle, infinity
Shu	'To raise', light, space, dryness
Sia	Insight, incarnation of intuitive consciousness
Smai	Union

T

Tawi	Two lands
Tama-re	Tamerri / name of Ancient Egypt/Afrika: 'land of the sun'
Tama-rean	Ancient Afrikan
Tama-reyaat	Ancient Egyptians
Tao	The way, balance
Tarug	Path / journey
Taruh	Hand
Tat	Low breathing
Taful	Prayer
Tehuti	Male personification of wisdom / master of divine words and sacred writings
Twa	People of Anu / The Twa Ptahrites/Pygmies

W

Waab	Spiritual priest

Y

Yaa	'Oh' summons, call upon

BIBLIOGRAPHY & RECOMMENDED READING

Afrika, L. O. (2004). *African Holistic Health*. Eworld Inc.

Ashby, M. (2006). *The African Origins of Hatha Yoga: And its Ancient Mystical Teaching*.

Ashby, M. (2005). *The African Origins: African Origins of African Civilization, Mystic Religion, Yoga Mystical: Volume 1*.

Ashby, M. (2005). *The African Origins: The African Origins of Western Civilization, Religion, and Philosophy: Volume 2*.

Ashby, M. (2005). *Egyptian Yoga: The Philosophy of Enlightenment: Volume 1*.

Bose, N.K. (1994). *The Structure of Hindu Society*. Sangam Books Ltd.

Castaneda, C. (1991). *The Fire from Within*. Simon & Schuster.

Castaneda, C. (1990). *The Teachings of Don Juan: A Yaqui Way of Knowledge*. Penguin.

Chandler, W. B. (2000). *Ancient Future: The Teachings and Prophetic Wisdom of the Seven Hermetic Laws of Ancient Egypt*. Black Classic Press.

Chung, T. C. (ed), (1992), trans by Kiang, K. K. *The Book of Zen: Freedom of The Mind (Asiapac Comic Series)*. Asiapac Books.

Easwaran, E. (2007). *The Bhagavad Gita (Classic of Indian Spirituality) (Easwaran's Classics of Indian Spirituality)*. Nilgiri Press.

Fuller, N. (1984). *The united independent compensatory code/system/concept: A textbook/workbook for thought, speech and/or action, for victims of racism (white supremacy)*. S.N.

Hotep, H. 'Solar Biology or Lunar Astrology'. Accessible, only in part, at https://www.scribd.com/doc/169540333/Hathor-Solar-Biology-Lunar-Astrology.

Karade, B. I. (1994) *The Handbook of Yoruba Religious Concepts*. Red Wheel/Weiser.

Karenga, M. (1989). *Selections from the Husia: Sacred Wisdom from Ancient Egypt*. University of Sankore Press.

King, R. (2012). *African Origin of Biological Psychiatry*.

King, R. (2012). *Melanin: A Key to Freedom*.

Kush, -K, I. (2014). *What They Never Told You in History Class*. Eworld Inc.

Liezi (1991), trans. by Kiang, K. K. *Sayings of Lie Zi: The Taoist Who Rides the Wind*. Bk.1. Singapore; Asiapac.

Massey, G. (1907). *Egyptian Book of the Dead and the Mysteries of Amenta*. London; T. Fisher Unwin.

Ra Un Nefer Amen (1990). Metu Neter Vol .1: *The Great Oracle of Tehuti and the Egyptian System of Spiritual Cultivation*. Kamit Pubns.

Rogers, J. A. (1995). 1*00 Amazing Facts About the Negro with Complete Proof: A Short Cut to the World History of the Negro*. Helga M. Rogers.

Sertima, I. V. (1988). *African Presence in Early Asia*. Transaction Publishers.

Siculus, D. (1933). *The Library of History, Vol 1 [online]*. Accessed on 3rd February 2021 at https://www.hup.harvard.edu/catalog.php?isbn=9780674993075#:~:text=Diodorus%20Siculus%2C%20Greek%20historian%20of,and%20history%20to%2054%20BCE.

Tzu, L. (2005) trans by Addiss, S. and Lombardo, S. *Tao Te Ching*. Hackett Publishing Co. Volney,C.F. (1999). *The Ruins of Empires*. US; Black Classic Press.

Wilson, A. N. (1993). *The Falsification of Afrikan Consciousness: Eurocentric History, Psychiatry and the Politics of White Supremacy (Awis Lecture Series)*. Afrikan World Infosystems.

Yamamoto, T. (2005). *Hagakure: Book of the Samurai*. Accessed on 17th February 2021 at http://3yryua3n3eu3i4gih2iopzph.wpengine.netdna-cdn.com/wp-content/uploads/2016/07/pdf/hagakure.pdf

York, M. Z. (1992). *The Sacred Records Of Neter: Aaferti Atum-Re*.

For further reading about black civilization and life in India between 10,000 BC to 1700 BC, see:

Barton, P. A. (2000). *Susu Economics: The History of Pan-African (Black) Trade, Commerce, Money and Wealth Part 1*. **Author House.**

Houston, D. D. (2014). *Wonderful Ethiopians of the Ancient Cushite Empire*. **Black Classic Press.**

Milton Keynes UK
Ingram Content Group UK Ltd.
UKHW050358261023
431322UK00004B/38